Total Health
Handbook

Total Health Handbook

Your Complete Wellness Resource

ALLAN MAGAZINER, D.O.

KENSINGTON BOOKS
http://www.kensingtonbooks.com

This publication and product is designed to provide accurate and authoritative information with regard to the subject matter covered. The purchase of this publication does not create a doctor-patient relationship between the purchaser and the author, nor should the information contained in this book be considered specific medical advice with respect to a specific patient and/or a specific condition. In the event the purchaser desires to obtain specific medical advice or other information concerning a specific person, condition, or situation, the services of a competent professional should be sought.

The author and publisher specifically disclaim any liability, loss, or risk, personal or otherwise, that is or may be incurred as a consequence, directly or indirectly, of the use and application of any of the information contained in this book.

KENSINGTON BOOKS are published by

Kensington Publishing Corp.
850 Third Avenue
New York, NY 10022

Kensington and the K logo Reg. U.S. Pat. & TM Off.

ISBN 1-57566-483-6

First Kensington Trade Paperback Printing: February, 2000
10 9 8 7 6 5 4 3 2 1

Printed in the United States of America

This book is dedicated to my mother and father, Mary and Irvin, for their lifelong inspiration and support; to my wife, Suzanne, for her enthusiasm and continued encouragement; to my wonderful children, who have given me a new perspective on the meaning of life; and finally, to my nephew, Erik, whose life was taken too soon. His valiant battle with leukemia invigorated my quest to find additional paths leading to physical and spiritual well-being.

ACKNOWLEDGMENTS

I would like to acknowledge the invaluable contributions of my illustrious colleagues who were pioneers in the field of environmental, nutritional, and preventive medicine. I extend my deepest gratitude to Jonathan V. Wright, M.D., and William J. Rea, M.D., who through postgraduate fellowship training imparted to me their vast knowledge, experience, and insight. Thanks must go to my sister Badiene for her tireless efforts in helping this educational guide come to fruition, Donna Levin for her valued help in editing, Cheryl Clerico for her preliminary work, and Evelyn Moriarty and Gayle Cohen for their assistance. Special thanks also go to my staff and patients at Magaziner Center for Wellness and Anti-Aging Medicine for their continued patience and support; to my agent, Maureen Walters; and to Paul Dinas, Richard Ember, Allan Graubard, Lee Heiman, and the rest of the staff at Kensington Publishing Corporation.

Contents

PREFACE

I have written this book to provide the tools needed to empower the reader to take responsibility for his or her own health and become an active participant in making the necessary lifestyle changes for achieving this goal. Through my years of practice, it became apparent to me that a better informed patient was more likely to make the commitment required to promote personal well-being. This up-to-date, practical, and comprehensive guide is designed to be a companion to assist you in following the recommendations of your health-care practitioner.

The material contained in this manual is information that my patients and I perceive as the most important to provide a sound foundation for natural healing. Many of the charts have been adapted from books, articles, newsletters, and handouts from my esteemed colleagues. This concise and easy-to-read book provides information in a variety of areas including diet, nutrition, wholesome foods, exercise, vitamins, minerals, herbal therapies, allergies, and environmental issues.

Although the traditional medical model focuses on protocols related to medication, surgery, chemotherapy, or radiation, I believe that we need to keep an open mind and go beyond the limitations of standard protocols when conventional medicine fails. In sharing this expanded approach, I hope this guide will assist you to incorporate newer ideas in your quest for achieving optimum health.

What Is the Purpose of This Handbook?

In my nearly twenty years of clinical experience, I have noted that patients have a need for further education. After treating over 10,000 patients and supervising more than 50,000 chelation treatments, it became evident to me that in order to take charge of their own health, patients need more in-depth knowledge to be able to heal themselves with the guidance of a doctor. This handbook provides tools to help you heal yourself and to further implement and follow up on your doctor's advice to enhance the doctor's treatment. I have been fortunate enough to have been trained by, and to have associated with, some of the world's leading authorities in nutrition, preventive and environmental medicine.

This handbook was written to fill a void in the field of nutrition and natural healing and to provide many answers to the most common questions you may have regarding your health. *Total Health Handbook* blends my clinical experience in successfully treating thousands of patients along with the latest research advances in alternative and complementary medicine.

Part I

FOOD, NUTRITION, AND DIETS

CHAPTER 1

Vital Nutrients

The doctor of the future will give no medicine but will interest his patients in the care of the human frame, in diet, and in the cause and prevention of disease.... The physician of tomorrow will be the nutritionist of today.

—Thomas Edison

Proper nutrition can prevent and treat numerous illnesses. Seven out of ten leading causes of death have a link to inappropriate food and alcohol intake. Many chronic illnesses can be prevented or treated by modifying your diet and lifestyle. Becoming ill as you progress through middle-age and your elderly years is not inevitable. Taking control and responsibility for your own health is absolutely essential, and the foods that you eat and the nutrients that you consume are of utmost importance. Furthermore, with proper nutrition, millions of dollars in national health-care expenditures could be saved. The evidence in favor of nutritional supplements and their ability to protect against chronic diseases continues to mount.

Proper nutrition includes a balance of vitamins, minerals, enzymes, amino acids, and essential fatty acids, all of which are the crucial building blocks used by all cells. Wholesome nutrition is required to effect growth, repair damaged tissues, and keep our bodies in a healthy state.

What's Wrong with the American Diet?

TOO MUCH:

- Total fat
- Saturated fat
- Cholesterol
- Alcohol
- Sugar
- Processed food

- Fried food
- Salt
- Calories
- Food preservatives and additives
- Artificial flavorings and colorings

TOO LITTLE:

- Fresh fruit and vegetables
- Variety of food

- Whole grains, beans, and legumes
- Fiber

Environmental factors such as nutrient-deficient soil, pesticides, and pollution can affect the quality of our food. Preservatives, colorings, and flavor enhancers also change the quality of the food we ingest. Furthermore, processing, storing, and transporting food can also deplete its nutritional value. All these factors lend greater support for the importance of eating high-quality, nutrient-dense foods that are loaded with important vitamins, minerals, antioxidants, and fiber.

Research has indicated that on any given day:

- 22 percent eat no vegetables at all.
- 45 percent have no fruit at all.
- Only 27 percent consume three or more vegetables.
- Only 29 percent consume two or more servings of fruit.
- Only 9 percent meet the USDA minimum recommendations of eating at least five servings of fruit and vegetables per day.

Vitamins for Vitality

Vitamins are organic compounds that are found in the foods we eat or that may be manufactured from our intestinal bacteria. They are involved in virtually every bodily function. Vitamins are either water soluble or fat soluble. The fat-soluble vitamins include vitamins A, E, D, and K while the water-soluble vitamins consist of a variety of B vitamins, vitamin C, and beta-carotene. While we should be eating fresh, wholesome foods whenever possible to get the majority of our vitamins, the reality is that the average American is eating a vitamin-deficient diet. Therefore, it may be advisable to supplement your diet with appropriate vitamin and mineral supplements. Furthermore, there is now substantial evidence that supplementation can help prevent several chronic diseases from arising in the first place such as heart disease, osteoporosis, and some forms of cancer. Page 12 will discuss the factors making nutritional supplements so important.

Water-soluble vitamins	Fat-soluble vitamins
• Are dissolved by body fluids and excreted through the urine. • Must be renewed regularly. • Have little chance of becoming toxic.	• Can be stored by the body's own fat cells and retained for use on demand. • Are not absorbed as easily as water-soluble supplements. • Can be overdosed.
Examples: Vitamin B_1 (thiamin) Vitamin B_2 (riboflavin) Vitamin B_3 (niacin, niacinamide) Vitamin B_5 (pantothenic acid) Vitamin B_6 (pyridoxine) Vitamin B_{12} (cobalamin) Vitamin C Beta-carotene Choline Inositol Biotin Folic acid PABA	*Examples:* Vitamin A Vitamin E (tocopherol) Vitamin D Vitamin K (menadione)

You are not what you eat—you are what you absorb from what you eat.

—Jeffrey Bland, Ph.D.

What Are the Major Vitamins, Their Functions, Their Sources, and the Effects of Deficiency?

Vitamin	Function	Food Source	Deficiency Predisposes to:
Vitamin A and beta-carotene	Potent antioxidant. Essential for immune system. Prevents night blindness. Vital for skin disorders and acne. Needed for tissue maintenance and repair.	Cheese Eggs Fish liver oils Green and yellow fruits and vegetables including: apricots asparagus broccoli carrots sweet potatoes squash Liver Milk	Skin disorders: acne, eczema, psoriasis Gum disorders Eye disorders: poor vision, night blindness, dry eyes Impaired growth and development Lowered resistance to infections
Vitamin C (ascorbic acid)	Key antioxidant. Stimulates immune system. Assists tissue repair and growth.	Citrus fruits Green vegetables Melons Berries Tomatoes	Scurvy Bleeding gums Pale skin Slow wound healing Lowered resistance to infection
Vitamin D	Prevents rickets and osteoporosis. Required for metabolism of calcium and phosphorus. Enhances immunity.	Egg yolk Fatty saltwater fish including salmon, tuna, herring Fish liver oils Vitamin D–fortified dairy products	Rickets (in children) Osteomalacia (softening and deformity of the bone in adults)
Vitamin E	Vital for red cell anticoagulation. Helps circulation. Cardio-protective effect. Aids tissue maintenance and repair. Potent antioxidant. Useful in treating PMS. Useful in treating fibrocystic breast disease. Enhances immunity.	Dark green, leafy vegetables Eggs Legumes Nuts Vegetable oils Wheat germ and whole grains	Vascular disorders Abnormal blood clotting Nervous system disorders
Vitamin K	Essential for blood clotting. Prevents osteoporosis.	Beef liver Green leafy vegetables	Abnormal blood clotting Bleeding problems
B_1 (thiamine)	Metabolizes fats, proteins, and carbohydrates. Essential for heart muscles, brain, and nervous system function.	Brewer's yeast Fish Meat Molasses Nuts Sunflower seeds Whole grains	Beriberi Indigestion Heart failure Muscle weakness

Vitamin	Function	Food Source	Deficiency Predisposes to:
B$_2$ (riboflavin)	Metabolizes fats, proteins, and carbohydrates. Builds body tissue. Builds red blood cells.	Blackstrap molasses Eggs Green leafy vegetables Legumes Nuts Poultry Fish Whole grains Beef	Sore throat and cracks in corners of the mouth Anemia Neuropathy Dry skin
B$_3$ (niacin/ niacinamide)	Metabolizes fats, proteins, and carbohydrates. Aids in digestion. Enhances HCL production. Regulates platelet aggregation and serum cholesterol. Helpful in treating osteoarthritis.	Eggs Legumes Meat Nuts Whole grains Poultry	Pellagra Diarrhea Swelling of mucous membranes
B$_6$ (pyridoxine)	Activates immune system. Assists digestion and enzyme activity. Aids metabolism of fatty acids and proteins. May protect against some forms of heart disease.	Avocados, bananas Beans, especially soy Egg yolks Peas Poultry and fish Walnuts, peanuts Whole grains Liver Milk	Decreased antibody production Dermatitis Rash and oral lesions Convulsions Nervousness Anemia
B$_{12}$ (cyanocobal-amin)	Aids digestion of fats, proteins, and carbohydrates. Assists formation of blood cells, RNA, and DNA. Vital for nervous system.	Animal foods Eggs Fermented soy products such as tofu and tempeh Fish, especially herring, mackerel Liver Milk products Nutritional yeast	Pernicious anemia Insomnia Peripheral neuropathy
Folic acid (folate)	Metabolizes amino acids. Vital for blood cell formation. Needed for healthy cell division and replication. Aids in production of hydrochloric acid, hemoglobin, and collagen. Assists B$_{12}$ utilization. Protects against spina bifida and other neural tube defects. May prevent heart disease. May protect against colon polyps.	Beef Bran Chicken liver Green leafy vegetables Lamb Legumes Pork Whole wheat Yeast	Anemia Increases risk of birth defects Mouth lesions

Vitamin	Function	Food Source	Deficiency Predisposes to:
B$_5$ (Pantothenic acid)	Metabolizes fats, proteins, and carbohydrates. Potent antioxidant. Assists nerve transmission. Aids adrenal gland function. Helps production of red blood cells.	All plant and animal products, especially organ meats Fresh vegetables Whole wheat Beans Saltwater fish Eggs	Insomnia Nausea
Biotin	Metabolizes proteins, fats, and carbohydrates. Synthesis of essential fatty acids.	Dark green vegetables Egg yolks Liver, kidney Milk Most fish, especially sardines Soybeans Whole grains	Anemia Depression Hair loss Brittle nails Dry skin
Choline and inositol	Metabolism, absorption, and utilization of cholesterol and fat. Lecithin synthesis. Brain neurotransmitter.	Whole grains Fruits Milk Organ meats Vegetables Egg yolks Soybeans	
PABA (para-aminobenzoic acid)	Aids in metabolism of protein and folic acid. Natural sunscreen.	Liver Kidney Molasses Dark green vegetables Whole grains Eggs Yogurt	
Bioflavonoids	Enhances capillary strength. Assists utilization of vitamin C.	Cabbage Cherries, Plums, Grapes Oranges, Grapefruit, Parsley	Slow healing Petechia (small "blood blisters") Broken blood vessels Bruising

Marvelous Minerals: From Boron to Zinc!

Minerals are essential for maintaining a healthy body. They act as cofactors for various biochemical and enzymatic reactions. Cofactors are substances which facilitate or assist metabolic processes such as bowel movements, sweating, heart rhythm, blood pressure control, glucose metabolism, and muscle contractions.

Minerals are obtained through a variety of foods and are utilized in various functions. Minerals are not manufactured by the body itself. Therefore, it is crucial that we ingest minerals through a variety of nutritious foods and through supplements to obtain the proper mineral balance.

I have found that more than 50 percent of my patients are actually deficient in at least one mineral, and several are deficient in two or more key minerals. Magnesium, zinc, and chromium, in particular, are three of the minerals that are frequently measured to be sub-optimal or deficient in patients that I treat for chronic conditions. I believe that this is due to the fact that most Americans are not eating fresh, unprocessed, nutrient-rich foods and so many are taking medications on a regular basis, which contribute to their deficiencies. More about medications will be discussed on pages 19–24.

What Are the Most Important Minerals, Their Functions, Their Sources, and the Effects of Deficiency?

Mineral	Function	Food Source	Deficiency Predisposes to:
Boron	Increases bone density in menopausal women.	Apples Peas Dark green vegetables Grapes	Osteoporosis
Calcium	Strengthens formation of bones and teeth. Regulates muscle contractions, hormones, and nerve impulses. Assists blood clotting.	Dairy foods Green leafy vegetables Nuts and seeds Salmon, sardines Tofu (soybean curd)	Osteoporosis Osteoarthritis Muscle cramps Insomnia
Chromium	Metabolizes glucose, fatty acids, and cholesterol. Assists insulin regulation.	Beans Black pepper Brewer's yeast Cheese Meat Mushrooms Peanuts Whole grains	Glucose intolerance
Copper	Necessary for bone and blood formation. Needed for maintenance of connective tissue. Required for formation of red blood cells. May lower cholesterol.	Avocado Cauliflower Dried beans and peas Green leafy vegetables Legumes Nuts Shellfish, especially oysters Whole grains	High blood cholesterol Anemia Arrhythmia

Mineral	Function	Food Source	Deficiency Predisposes to:
Fluorine	Needed to maintain strong teeth and strong bones.	Fluoridated water Seafood	Weak bones and teeth
Iodine	Aids thyroid function. Prevents goiter development. Promotes energy metabolism. Enhances hair, nails, and skin.	Iodized salt Kelp Saltwater fish Seafood Seaweed	Enlarged thyroid gland (goiter) Mental retardation Obesity
Iron	Essential for hemoglobin production. Assists energy production. Vital for healthy immune function.	Eggs Fish Green leafy vegetables Legumes Meat Poultry Liver Molasses Whole grains	Anemia Recurrent infections Glossitis Stomatitis Fatigue
Magnesium	Vital for heart and muscle function. Essential for bone formation. Facilitates enzyme systems.	Bananas Dried beans and peas Green vegetables Seafood Whole grains and nuts	Leg cramps Coronary vasospasm Hypertension Arrhythmia Muscle fatigue Insomnia Anxiety
Manganese	Essential for normal bones and cartilage formation. Needed for healthy nerves. Necessary for metabolism of proteins, cholesterol, and fats. Needed for sex hormone formation. Activates enzymes for vitamins C, B_{12} and biotin.	Avocado Celery Dried beans and peas Egg yolks Liver and kidney Nuts and seeds Pineapple Seaweed Whole grains	Brittle bones Carbohydrate intolerance Abnormal glucose levels
Molybdenum	Assists iron utilization. Facilitates carbohydrate and fat metabolism. Useful in sulfite metabolism.	Dried beans and peas Green leafy vegetables Meat, especially lamb Whole grains	Asthma Increased risk of esophageal and stomach cancer
Phosphorus	Necessary for metabolism of calcium, vitamins, fats, proteins, and carbohydrates. Vital for healthy bones and teeth. Assists tissue growth and repair. Facilitates energy production.	Dairy products Eggs Legumes Meat, poultry, and fish Nuts and seeds Whole grains	Gum disorders Weak bones

Mineral	Function	Food Source	Deficiency Predisposes to:
Potassium	Regulates water and sodium balance. Needed for nervous system, hormone secretion, and muscle contractions. Helps regulate blood pressure. Controls heart activity.	Dairy foods Fish Fruit, especially bananas, citrus, and apricots Legumes Meat, poultry Sunflower seeds Vegetables, especially potatoes Whole grains	Heart arrhythmia Muscle weakness Lethargy
Selenium	Vital antioxidant. Necessary for tissue elasticity. Important for growth and fertility. Prevents heart disease. Protects against cancer. Assists immune response.	Broccoli Garlic Meats, liver, kidney Mushrooms Seafood Wheat germ Whole grains	Has been implicated in development of cancer and heart failure
Sodium	Regulates fluid balance.	Salt	
Vanadium	Active in lipid metabolism. Enhances cholesterol metabolism. Helps glucose utilization.	Buckwheat Eggs Oats Parsley Soybeans	High cholesterol Diabetes
Zinc	Vital for burn and wound healing. Active in production of enzymes. Promotes insulin production. Protects liver from chemical damage. Activates immune system. Involved in protein metabolism.	Dried beans and peas Eggs Legumes Meats and poultry Seafood Soybeans Sunflower seeds Whole grains	Stunting of growth in children Poor healing and wound repair Inefficient immune response Poor sense of smell and taste Night blindness

Who Needs Supplements?

It has been estimated that nearly 50 percent of the general population take vitamin supplements on a regular basis. Eating a well-balanced, varied diet is essential to avoid vitamin and mineral deficiencies and their accompanying symptoms. The fact is, however, that most Americans are simply not consuming the Recommended Daily Allowances for most vitamins and minerals on a regular basis through diet alone. Therefore, more people are turning to dietary supplements to help assist their nutritional needs and replace the missing nutrients.

More recently, nutritional supplements have also been associated with protection against heart disease, stroke, cancer, osteoporosis, memory loss, chronic infections, and may even slow down the aging process. The key, however, is finding out which supplements you really need, how much to take, when to take them, in what form, and what brand. These issues are quite complex and need to be individualized from one person to another.

Our inability to effectively digest, absorb, and utilize our food may increase the need for nutritional supplements. Medications and illness may also alter our nutritional needs. In addition, environmental factors, smoking, and the ingestion of excess alcohol and coffee may deplete various nutrients and increase the need for supplements. High levels of stress may also deplete certain nutrients and increase the need for supplemental vitamins, minerals, and amino acids.

WHICH FACTORS MAKE NUTRITIONAL SUPPLEMENTS NECESSARY?

- Insufficient food intake or poor diet
- Malabsorption or poor assimilation
- Specific genetic or acquired vitamin dependency
- Biochemical individuality or uniqueness
- Extra needs of the elderly
- Pregnancy, lactation, or heavy menstrual bleeding
- Recovery from traumatic injuries and surgery
- Deficiencies due to prescription or over-the-counter medication
- Detrimental effects of cigarette smoking or exposure to secondhand smoke
- Deficiencies due to alcohol abuse
- Extra needs of those exercising heavily

Natural Versus Synthetic?

Natural and synthetic vitamins are chemically similar in structure and similar in the functions that they perform. However, it is advisable to purchase natural supplements whenever possible. In the case of vitamin E, for example, natural forms have been found to be more bioavailable or absorbable than synthetic forms. Furthermore, chemically sensitive individuals may have adverse reactions to the fillers and binders used in synthetic supplements.

Natural supplements are extracted from food sources and consist of nutrients and other constituents that are more likely to be found in nature. Synthetic supplements, which are chemically manufactured in a lab, are less likely to contain naturally occurring enzymes or minerals.

Attempt to avoid supplements with sugar, artificial dyes, or preservatives. Check labels on natural products for guarantees such as "No sugar, starch, salt, milk, yeast, wheat, corn, preservatives, artificial colors or flavors."

Can Antioxidants Slow the Aging Process?

Antioxidants are nutrients that seek out free radicals and neutralize their damaging effects before they can do damage to cellular structures. If left unchecked, free radicals can damage the body's cells and tissues. Free radicals are chemical compounds produced in the body as a result of exposure to radiation, toxic metals, pesticides, environmental pollutants, and naturally occurring biochemical processes. Free radicals have been implicated in contributing to common health problems such as cancer, diabetes, heart attacks, strokes, premature aging, macular degeneration, and cataracts. Antioxidants play a major role in maintaining health, vigor, and avoiding premature aging.

As you get older, you may have a greater need for specific antioxidants. Even though you should do your best to obtain them from the foods you eat, supplements containing antioxidants are also a powerful way of preventing free radicals from wreaking havoc and damaging your cells.

WHAT ARE THE BENEFITS OF ANTIOXIDANTS?

- May reduce death rates by 50 percent.
- May reduce cancer rates by 13 percent.
- May reduce skin cancer by 70 percent.
- May reduce heart attacks by 50 percent.
- May reduce strokes by 50 percent.
- May reduce risk of cataracts by 27 to 36 percent.
- May boost cancer survival rates by 50 percent.
- May boost immunity by 50 percent.
- May reduce infections by 50 percent.

What Are the Most Important Antioxidants?

ANTIOXIDANTS AND THEIR FUNCTION

Potent Antioxidants	Function
Vitamin C	Prevents heart disease, stimulates immune system, necessary for tissue repair, protects against cancer.
Vitamin E	Prevents heart disease, stimulates immune system, improves oxygen utilization, protects against cancer.
Beta-carotene	Enhances immune system, protects against environmental chemicals, antiviral properties, protects against cancer.
CoQ_{10}	Increases oxygen to the tissues, protects the heart, protects against cancer, assists ability of cells to make energy.
Selenium	Protects against cancer, assists immune system, necessary for elasticity of skin, protects against affects of ozone radiation.
Glutathione (GSH)	Assists liver detoxification, enhances immune response, protects against cancer, protects against macular degeneration and cataracts.

What Are the Main Dietary Sources of Antioxidants?

Fruits and vegetables are an excellent source of fiber and antioxidant vitamins A and C, which help protect against cancer, heart disease, and other degenerative diseases. Vitamin E, another potent antioxidant, can be found in nuts, seeds, and oils. The following table lists dietary sources of three significant antioxidants: vitamin A, vitamin C, and vitamin E.

Truly, the vegetable kingdom contains our best medicines.
—Henry G. Bieler, M.D.

DIETARY SOURCES OF ANTIOXIDANT VITAMINS

Source	Serving Size	Amount
Vitamin A		
Apricots, dried	½ cup	7,085 IU
Bran, wheat	1 cup	1,650 IU
Broccoli, cooked	1 cup	3,800 IU
Cantaloupe	¼	3,400 IU
Carrots, cooked	1 cup	15,750 IU
Carrots, raw	1	11,000 IU
Endive, raw	1 cup	1,650 IU
Mango	1	11,090 IU
Parsley, chopped	1 cup	5,100 IU
Peaches	1	1,330 IU
Prunes, dried	1 cup	2,580 IU
Spinach, cooked	1 cup	14,850 IU
Squash, winter	1 cup	8,610 IU
Tomato, raw	1	1,350 IU
Watermelon	1 slice	3,540 IU
Vitamin C		
Acerola juice	1 cup	3,872 mg
Black currants	1 cup	200 mg
Broccoli, cooked	1 cup	140 mg
Brussels sprouts	1 cup	135 mg
Cauliflower	1 cup	69 mg
Grapefruit	1	76 mg
Grapefruit juice	1 cup	95 mg
Guava	1	242 mg
Lettuce	1 cup	75 mg
Mango	1	81 mg
Mustard greens	1 cup	117 mg
Orange	1	66 mg
Parsley	1 cup	103 mg
Peppers, green	1 cup	103 mg
Strawberries	1 cup	88 mg
Tomato, raw	1	34 mg
Watermelon	1 slice	42 mg
Vitamin E		
Almonds	3.5 oz	41 IU
Margarine, hard	3.5 oz	16 IU
Margarine, soft	3.5 oz	21 IU
Mayonnaise	3.5 oz	19 IU
Peanut oil	3.5 oz	28 IU
Peanuts, dry roasted	3.5 oz	11 IU
Safflower oil	3.5 oz	59 IU
Soybean oil	3.5 oz	12 IU
Sunflower oil	3.5 oz	73 IU
Sunflower seeds	3.5 oz	74 IU
Wheat germ oil	3.5 oz	178 IU

What Produce Is Highest in Fiber, Vitamin A, and Vitamin C?

The following table identifies foods highest in antioxidant vitamins C and A and fiber, which may be helpful in cancer prevention. Incorporating these foods into your diet is absolutely essential, especially if you have a history of previous cancer or if there is a strong family history of cancer. Try to become more familiar with these foods since they have so many protective effects.

ANTICANCER PRODUCE

Vegetable	High in Vitamin C	High in Vitamin A	Moderate/High in Fiber
Asparagus	✓	✓	✓
Beets	✓	✓	✓
Broccoli*	✓	✓	✓
Brussels sprouts*	✓		
Cabbage*	✓		✓
Cauliflower*	✓		
Chard		✓	
Collard	✓	✓	
Corn			✓
Dandelion		✓	
Eggplant			✓
Kale	✓	✓	✓
Kohlrabi	✓		
Mustard	✓	✓	
Parsley		✓	
Peas	✓		
Peppers, green	✓		✓
Peppers, red	✓	✓	
Romaine lettuce		✓	
Spinach	✓		✓
Sweet potatoes		✓	✓
Tomatoes	✓	✓	✓
Turnip	✓	✓	✓
Watercress	✓	✓	
Winter squash	✓	✓	✓

*In addition to their high vitamin content, these cruciferous vegetables contain substances called indoles, which deactivate carcinogens and block them from damaging cells. Broccoli sprouts are particularly high in the indole known as sulfurophane, which may be able to block tumor cells from forming. Recently, one particular indole, known as indole-3-carbinol, has been found to reverse abnormal, pre-cancerous cervical cells called cervical dysplasia. These indoles detoxify carcinogens and alter estrogen metabolism. In general, cruciferous vegetables such as Brussels sprouts, cabbage, and broccoli are thought to be protective against colon, lung, and breast cancer.

Phytochemicals: Fantastic Fruits and Vitalizing Vegetables!

Phytochemicals occur in plants and have the ability to act as potent antioxidants. Researchers theorize that phytochemicals, a component of fruits and vegetables, can prevent disease and act therapeutically when ingested. Phytochemicals may prevent and reverse cancers, including melanoma, and reduce the incidence of breast and prostate cancer. Some phytochemicals have been shown to prevent heart disease. Listed below are some beneficial chemicals and the various foods in which they can be found, as well as their possible benefits. I strongly recommend that you try to incorporate many of these phytochemical-containing foods into your diet.

PROTECTIVE PHYTOCHEMICALS AND THEIR BENEFITS

Phytochemical	Found in	Possible Benefit
Allium	Garlic, leeks, onions	Breaks down cancer-causing chemicals. May lower blood cholesterol and risk of heart disease.
Carnosol	Rosemary	May inhibit growth of some tumors.
Carotenoids	Tomatoes, watermelon, grapefruit	Prevents lung cancer.
Capsaicin	Hot peppers	Protects DNA from carcinogens. Acts as an antioxidant.
Coumarins	Citrus fruit, tomatoes, nuts, beans, grains	Stimulates anticancer enzymes. Prevents blood clotting.
Flavonoids	Citrus fruit, tomatoes, berries, peppers carrots, onions, kale, grape skin, red wine	Prevents cancer-promoting hormones from attaching themselves to normal cells. Inhibits enzymes responsible for cancer cell metastasis. Prevents heart disease by preventing oxidation of LDL cholesterol.
Genistein	Peas, lentils, soybeans	Inhibits estrogen-promoted cancers. Protects against osteoporosis and menopausal symptoms.
Indoles	Broccoli, cabbage, kale, Brussels sprouts	Protects against breast, ovarian, and prostate cancer. May boost immune function.
Isoflavones	Soy products (tofu, tempeh, miso)	Inhibits breast, ovarian, and endometrial cancers. Protects against osteoporosis and heart disease.
Isothiocyanates (sulforaphane)	Broccoli, cabbage, mustard, horseradish	Stimulates anticancer enzymes and protects against breast cancer.
Lignans	Flaxseed, barley, wheat	Acts as an antioxidant. Stimulates enzymes that detoxify cancer cells.
Lycopene	Tomatoes, red grapefruit, watermelons, strawberries	Acts as an antioxidant. Protects against cardiovascular disease and cervical, colon, and prostate cancer.
S-allycysteine	Garlic, onions, chives, strawberries	Stimulates anticancer enzymes. Blocks formation of nitrite in stomach.
Saponins	Soybeans, lentils	Cuts the spread of cancer cells in the colon. Lowers cholesterol.
Triterpenoids	Licorice root, citrus fruit	Inhibits hormone-dependent steps in tumor formation.

What Are the Smartest, Healthiest Ways to Eat Your Vegetables?

Try to eat at least three to five servings of vegetables per day. The key point is simple: "Eat your vegetables." You should eat a variety of different vegetables, and they can be prepared in various ways. Consider raw vegetables when possible along with steamed, cooked, blanched, or even pureed as in the case of tomato sauce. Vegetables are packed with important antioxidants, phytochemicals, and large amounts of fiber.

Food	Power Ingredients	Preparation	Health Hints
Beans and legumes	Folic acid Fiber Phytochemicals 　Protease inhibitors 　Saponins 　Isoflavins	Phytochemicals keep their potency during cooking whether the legumes or beans are fresh or canned. They are still active in soybean products such as tofu, tempeh, and soy milk.	Sprinkle vitamin C–rich bean sprouts on salads, soups, or sandwiches.
Broccoli	Vitamin C Folic acid Calcium Fiber Phytochemicals 　Indoles 　Isothiocyanates 　Carotenoids	Eat raw or steamed.	Eat the leaves for extra calcium and the stalks for added fiber and vitamin C. Peel the stalks and slice widthwise. Cook them quickly along with the florets.
Cabbage	Vitamin C Fiber Phytochemicals 　Indoles 　Isothiocyanates 　Carotenoids	Eat raw in salads. Light and air deplete vitamin potency. Shred just before serving to minimize exposure.	Choose bok choy, a Chinese cabbage that's higher in phytochemicals and calcium than either red or green cabbage.
Carrots	Vitamin C Calcium Fiber Phytochemicals 　Carotenoids	Eat raw or steamed. To facilitate absorption of carotenoids, drizzle with vegetable or nut oil.	Prepeeled and baby carrots have the lowest levels of nutrients!
Greens 　Mustard 　Collard 　Turnip	Vitamin C Calcium Folic acid Phytochemicals 　Indoles 　Carotenoids	Even though eating them raw may be healthiest, these veggies are too tough to consume uncooked. Steaming is the best way to cook them to preserve the nutrients.	The deeper the color, the more healthful the vegetable.

Food	Power Ingredients	Preparation	Health Hints
Onions	Vitamin C Fiber Phytochemicals Allium compounds Flavonoids	Eat raw, roast, or sauté quickly. Chop or crush to release phytochemicals.	Red-skinned onions have the highest levels of certain flavonoids.
Sweet potatoes	Vitamin C Fiber Phytochemicals Flavonoids Carotenoids	Scrub well and bake in the oven.	Eat the skin! It is especially high in fiber and nutrients.
Tomatoes	Vitamin C Fiber Phytochemicals Coumarins Carotenoids Lycopene	Eat raw, puree and drink as a juice, or simmer in homemade sauces.	When possible, choose vine-ripened varieties. They absorb more nutrients when left to mature on the vine. The acidity of tomatoes helps them retain vitamin C during cooking.

> **TIP**
>
> Chop onions and tomatoes together with fresh cilantro to make a delicious salsa. It's a tasty treat and is filled with healthy phytochemicals.

Do Medications Deplete Your Nutrients?

While medications may be necessary for maintaining health and treating illness, they can also deplete the body of important nutrients. The medications you take may be causing deficiencies of specific nutrients by:

- Increasing urinary excretion of nutrients.
- Blocking absorption of the nutrients.
- Binding to the nutrients and inactivating them.
- Using up nutrients more rapidly.
- Destroying nutrients.
- Increasing the loss of nutrients through the stool.

I have seen an all-too-common problem where physicians prescribe diuretics for their patients in an effort to treat high blood pressure. These drugs often deplete potassium from your body and your prescribing physician rightfully recommends taking potassium along with it. However, another mineral, magnesium, is lost upon taking most diuretics and this mineral is frequently not replaced. As mentioned previously, magnesium is so important for the cardiovascular system. Even though you may be on a diuretic to help treat your hypertension, your blood pressure may not improve if your magnesium is being depleted!

If you are taking any of the following medications, you are at a greater risk for developing a vitamin or mineral deficiency and may require a supplement program.

Medication Class	Drugs Generic/Proprietary	Vitamins and Minerals Depleted
Antibiotics	Neomycin Tetracycline Gentamicin	Vitamin B_2, biotin, folic acid, niacin, vitamins C and D, calcium, iron, magnesium, potassium, zinc
Anticoagulant	Coumadin	(Avoid vitamin K)
Anticonvulsants	Dilantin Mysoline	Vitamins D and K, folic acid, calcium
Anti-Inflammatory	Aspirin Azulfidine Colchicine Cortisone	Iron, vitamin C Folic acid Beta-carotene, B_{12}, sodium, potassium, fat, niacin, vitamins C, D, K, and B_6
Antimalarial	Chloroquine Pyrimethamine	Folic acid
Antiparkinson	Levodopa	Vitamin B_6
Antipsychotic	Thorazine Mellaril	Riboflavin, vitamins B_{12} and D, calcium
Antituberculosis	INH Rifampin	Vitamin B_6, niacin, vitamin D
Chemotherapy	Cisplatin Methotrexate Adriamycin	iron, magnesium, Vitamin B_{12}, folic acid, vitamin E
Cholesterol-lowering agents	Cholestyramine	Vitamins A, B_{12} and K, folic acid, iron, coQ_{10}
Diabetes	Glucophage	Vitamin B_{12}
Diuretic	Lasix Thiazides	Vitamins B_6 and C, magnesium, potassium, zinc
Gastrointestinal antacids	Maalox Mylanta	Vitamins A, B_1, B_2, and B_6, folic acid, calcium, copper, iron, phosphorus
Laxatives	Mineral oil	Beta-carotene, vitamins A, D, E, and K, calcium, potassium
H_2 blockers	Cimetidine Ranitidine	Vitamin B_{12}
Menopause	Prempro	Vitamins B_2, B_6, and B_{12}, folic acid, magnesium, zinc
Oral contraceptives	Estrogen Progestin	Vitamins B_1, B_2, B_3, B_6, B_{12}, and C, folic acid, calcium, magnesium, zinc (increases iron and copper levels)

How Do Medications Affect
Your Vitamin and Nutrient Status?

The following table indicates the vitamins and minerals depleted from different medications. You should be aware of these if you take drugs for a prolonged period of time.

Medication Class	Drugs Generic/Proprietary	Vitamins and Minerals Depleted
Cholesterol-lowering agents	Cholestyramine	Vitamin A and beta-carotene
Laxatives	Mineral oil	
Antacids	Maalox	
	Mylanta	
Anticonvulsants	Dilantin	Vitamin D
Cholesterol-lowering agents	Cholestyramine	
Antituberculous	Isoniazid	
	Rifampin	
Laxatives	Mineral oil	
Antibiotics	Neomycin	
	Tetracycline	
Anti-inflammatories	Cortisone	
Antipsychotic	Haldol	
	Mellaril	
	Thorazine	
Anticancer	Cisplatin	Vitamin E
	Methotrexate	
Cholesterol-lowering agents	Cholestyramine	
Laxatives	Mineral oil	
Antibiotic	Neomycin	Vitamin K
Anticonvulsant	Mysoline	
Anticoagulant	Coumadin	
Anti-inflammatory	Colchicine	
Cholesterol-lowering agents	Cholestyramine	
Laxatives	Mineral oil	
Antacids	Maalox	Vitamin B_1 (Thiamine)
	Mylanta	
Alcohol		
Oral contraceptives		
Antibiotics	Tetracycline	Vitamin B_2 (Riboflavin)
Antipsychotic	Chlorpromazine	
	Thorazine	
Antacids	Maalox	
	Mylanta	
Alcohol		
Diuretics		
Oral contraceptives		

Medication Class	Drugs Generic/Proprietary	Vitamins and Minerals Depleted
Antituberculous	Isoniazid	Vitamin B$_3$ (Niacin)
Rifampin		
Antacids	Maalox	
	Mylanta	
Alcohol		
Oral contraceptives		
Alcohol		
Antacids	Maalox	Vitamin B$_6$ (Pyridoxine)
Antihypertensive	Hydralazine	
Anti-inflammatory	Prednisone	
Antiparkinson	Levodopa	
Antituberculous	Isoniazid	
	Rifampin	
Gastrointestinal	Donnatal	
Menopause	Premarin	
Oral contraceptives		
Alcohol		
Anesthetics	Nitrous oxide	Vitamin B$_{12}$ (Cobalamin)
Antacids	Maalox	
	Mylanta	
Antibiotics	Neomycin	
	Tetracycline	
Anticholesterol	Cholestyramine	
Antihypertensive	Methyldopa	
Anti-inflammatory	Colchicine	
	Prednisone	
Antipsychotics	Haldol	
	Mellaril	
	Thorazine	
Diabetes	Glucophage	
Gastrointestinal	Cimetidine	
	Ranitidine	
Alcohol		
Antacids	Maalox	Folic acid
	Mylanta	
Antibiotics	Isoniazid	
	Rifampin	
	Trimethoprim	
Anticancer	Adriamycin	
	Cisplatin	
	Methotrexate	
Anticholesterol	Cholestyramine	
Anticonvulsants	Dilantin	
	Phenobarbital	
Anti-inflammatory	Aspirin	
	Azulfidine	
	Colchicine	
	Methotrexate	
	Prednisone	

Medication Class	Drugs Generic/Proprietary	Vitamins and Minerals Depleted
Antimalarials	Chloroquine	Folic acid (cont'd.)
Pyrimethamine		
Diuretics	Dyazide	
Gastrointestinal	Donnatal	
Menopause	Premarin	
Oral contraceptives		
Antacids	Maalox	Vitamin C (ascorbic acid)
	Mylanta	
Antibiotics	Tetracyline	
Anti-inflammatory	Aspirin	
	Indomethacin	
	Tylenol	
Diuretics	Lasix	
	Thiazides	
Oral contraceptives		
Tobacco		
Cholesterol-lowering agents	Lescol	CoQ_{10}
	Lipitor	
	Mevacor	
Antacids	Maalox	Calcium
	Mylanta	
Antibiotics	Tetracycline	
Anticholesterol	Cholestyramine	
Anticonvulsants	Dilantin	
	Phenobarbital	
Anti-inflammatory	Prednisone	
Gastrointestinal	Donnatal	
	Mineral oil	
Heart	Digoxin	
Oral contraceptives		
Antacids	Maalox	Iron
	Mylanta	
Antibiotics	Neomycin	
Anticancer	Cisplatin	
	Methotrexate	
Anticholesterol	Cholestyramine	
Anti-inflammatory	Aspirin	
	Colchicine	
	Indomethacin	
	Prednisone	

Medication Class	Drugs Generic/Proprietary	Vitamins and Minerals Depleted
Alcohol		Magnesium
Antibiotics	Gentamicin	
	Neomycin	
	Tetracycline	
Anticancer	Cisplatin	
	Methotrexate	
Anticonvulsants	Dilantin	
	Edecrin	
	Mysoline	
	Phenobarbital	
Anti-inflammatory	Colchicine	
	Methotrexate	
Diuretics	Lasix	
	Thiazides	
Heart	Digoxin	
Menopause	Premarin	
Oral contraceptives		
Antibiotics	Gentamicin	Potassium
	Tetracycline	
Anticonvulsants	Edecrin	
Laxatives	Mineral oil	
	Phenolphthalein	
Diuretics	Lasix	
	Thiazides	
Antibiotics	Neomycin	Sodium
Anticancer	Vincristine	
Antidepressant	Elavil	
Anti-inflammatory	Colchicine	
Diuretics	Captopril	
	Mannitol	
	Spironlactone	
	Thiazides	
Alcohol		Zinc
Anti-inflammatory	Penicillamine	
Diuretics		

In America, there are 400 deaths each day from the side effects of prescription medicine.
—U.S. News and World Report, December 1994

A Word about Calcium

Calcium is a vitally important mineral necessary for all tissue and metabolic functions. Most people fall short of consuming the recommended dietary allowances for calcium. To prevent calcium deficiency, ingest at least 1,000 mg per day. There may be greater needs for pregnant, lactating, or postmenopausal women. As you can see, milk is not the only source of calcium. If you avoid dairy products or are lactose intolerant, there are numerous other choices. The following list informs you of the best nondairy sources of calcium-rich foods. These foods are also rich in other key vitamins and minerals, which may benefit you more than simply drinking a glass of milk.

NONDAIRY FOODS HIGH IN CALCIUM

Almonds	English walnuts	Oranges	Kombu*
Apricots, dried	Fennel	Parsley	Nori*
Artichokes	Figs*	Parsnips	Wakame*
Beet greens	Filberts	Peas	Sesame seeds*
Black currants	Green snap beans	Peaches, dried	Shallots
Brazil nuts	Horseradish	Pecans	Shrimp
Broccoli	Hot red pepper, dry	Pinto beans	Soy milk*
Brussels sprouts	Kale*	Pistachio nuts	Soybeans*
Cabbage	Kelp	Prunes*	Spinach
Carrots	Kidney beans*	Pumpkins	Squash
Cashew nuts	Kohlrabi	Raisins	Sunflower seeds
Celery	Kumquats	Red beans	Swiss chard
Cheese	Leeks	Rhubarb	Tangerines
Chestnuts	Lentils*	Rice	Taro leaves and
Chickpeas	Lettuce	Rutabaga	stems
Chicory greens	Lima beans	Rye grain	Tofu*
Chinese cabbage	Macadamia nuts	Salmon	Turnips
Chives	Mung beans	Sardines (with	Turnip greens
Collards*	Mustard greens*	bones)*	Watercress
Dandelion greens	Mustard spinach	Sea vegetables	Wheat
Dates*	Okra	Agar*	White beans
Elderberry	Olives	Arame*	
Endive (escarole)	Onions, green	Dulce*	
		Hijiki*	

*Highest sources of calcium

CALCIUM CONTENT OF FOOD—FROM HIGHEST TO LOWEST

Food	Amount	Calcium (mg)
Sesame seeds	1 cup	1,050
Wakame	1 oz	350
Milk (2%)	1 cup	350
Collards	⅔ cup	320
Cheese, cheddar	1 oz slice	215
Kale	⅔ cup	180
Mustard greens	⅔ cup	170
Broccoli	1 medium stalk	158
Tofu	4 oz	150
Spinach	⅔ cup	110
Shrimp	3 oz	100
Swiss chard	⅔ cup	85
Cheese, cottage	3 oz	80
Cabbage	⅔ cup	45
Snap beans	⅔ cup	45
Eggs	1 (large)	25
Bread, whole wheat	1 slice	25
Rice	1 cup	20
Kidney beans (cooked)	⅓ cup	20
Chicken	4 oz	10
Hamburger	3 oz patty	10
Orange	1 (medium)	10

Source: U.S. Dept. of Agriculture: *Nutritive Value of American Foods.*

CHAPTER 2

Proteins, Amino Acids, and Enzymes

Let food be your medicine and medicine be your food.
—Hippocrates, the fifth-century B.C. doctor,
traditionally regarded as the "father of medicine"

Proteins are essential in building muscle and new tissues, and repairing damaged tissues and cells. They help maintain fluid balance and are an important source of energy. Proteins are formed when amino acids are grouped together. Both essential amino acids, those derived directly from food intake, and nonessential, those derived from the metabolism of other amino acids, are the necessary building blocks that make up all proteins. Protein intake should probably not make up more than 15 percent of your total calories, since too much protein can put extra stress on your kidneys and has also been associated with calcium loss from the bones. On the other hand, eating adequate protein is essential. Thus, the proper balance of protein is key.

Did You Know That Spinach Has More Protein Than Milk?

Many people have the misconception that they have to ingest large quantities of meat, poultry, or fish to receive adequate protein. Plant sources such as vegetables, legumes, grains, and fruit also provide a rich source of protein. They are lower in fat than meat, poultry, and fish, and can be used as a substitute for animal protein.

A wonderful plant-based source of protein can be derived by eating more soy products. Try to incorporate soybeans, soy milk, tofu (soybean curd), or tempeh into your diet.

Not only are these soy products high in protein, but they contain numerous phytochemicals which, as previously discussed on page 17, can protect you against heart disease, osteoporosis, and some forms of cancer. If you are not familiar with how to prepare these foods, I suggest purchasing a vegetarian cookbook or searching for a vegetarian cooking class. The table below lists various sources of protein not only from animal sources but from plant sources, as well. Keep in mind that the plant-based foods also have the advantage of being lower in calories, cholesterol, and fat than most animal protein. They are also higher in fiber.

PERCENTAGES OF CALORIES FROM PROTEIN

Legumes

Soybean sprouts	54
Mung bean sprouts	43
Soybean curd (tofu)	43
Soy flour	35
Soybeans	35
Soy sauce	33
Broad beans	32
Lentils	29
Split peas	28
Kidney beans	26
Navy beans	26
Lima beans	26
Garbanzo beans	23

Grains

Wheat germ	31
Wheat, hard red	17
Wild rice	16
Buckwheat	15
Oatmeal	15
Millet	12
Barley	11
Spaghetti	9
Brown rice	8

Meat, Poultry, and Fish

Pork chop	82
Chicken with skin	78
Sirloin steak	71
White tuna	67
Ground beef	62
Flounder	51

Nuts and Seeds

Pumpkin seeds	21
Peanuts	18
Sunflower seeds	17
Walnuts, black	13
Sesame seeds	13
Almonds	12
Cashews	12
Filberts	8

Dairy

Cheese pizza	33
Cottage cheese	31
Cheddar cheese	24
Milk	18

Vegetables

Spinach	49
New Zealand spinach	47
Watercress	46
Kale	45
Broccoli	45
Brussels sprouts	44
Turnip greens	43
Collards	43
Cauliflower	40
Mustard greens	39
Mushrooms	38
Chinese cabbage	34
Parsley	34
Lettuce	34
Green peas	30
Zucchini	28
Green beans	26
Cucumbers	24
Dandelion greens	24
Green pepper	22
Artichokes	22
Cabbage	22
Celery	21
Eggplant	21
Tomatoes	18
Onions	16
Beets	15
Pumpkin	12
Potatoes	11
Yams	8
Sweet potatoes	6

Fruits

	16
Lemons	10
Honeydew melon	9
Cantaloupe	8
Strawberry	8
Orange	8
Blackberry	8
Cherry	8
Apricot	8
Grape	8
Watermelon	7
Tangerine	6
Papaya	6
Peach	5
Pear	5
Banana	5
Grapefruit	3
Pineapple	1
Apple	

Source: *United States Department of Agriculture Handbook #456.*

How Can I Get Enough Protein Without Eating Meat?

Many people are concerned about a lack of protein when instituting a vegetarian diet. Your protein needs can be easily met by properly combining vegetarian foods. On a vegetarian diet, it is necessary to properly combine legumes, whole grains, and nuts and seeds. For example, legumes and grains when eaten together, combine to produce a complete protein. Whole grains when eaten with nuts and seeds, also combine to produce a complete protein, as do legumes, when combined with nuts and seeds.

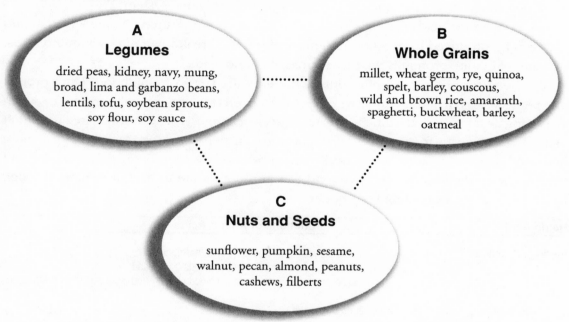

A
Legumes

dried peas, kidney, navy, mung, broad, lima and garbanzo beans, lentils, tofu, soybean sprouts, soy flour, soy sauce

B
Whole Grains

millet, wheat germ, rye, quinoa, spelt, barley, couscous, wild and brown rice, amaranth, spaghetti, buckwheat, barley, oatmeal

C
Nuts and Seeds

sunflower, pumpkin, sesame, walnut, pecan, almond, peanuts, cashews, filberts

Combine any two of the three groups below to obtain the essential amino acids necessary to form a complete protein.

SUGGESTED COMBINATIONS FOR FORMING COMPLETE PROTEINS

Combination A and B	Combination A and C	Combination B and C
• Rice with stir-fried tofu chunks	• Hummus dip with ground sesame seeds (gomasio)	• Whole grain cereal with pecans and walnuts
• Pea soup with whole grain rye bread	• Pureed mung beans with ground sunflower seeds	• Cooked oats with almond slivers
• Barley with kidney beans	• Garbanzo-cashew dip	• Rice with pine nuts (pignoli)
• Quinoa and lentils	• Tofu spread with chopped almonds	• Whole grain bread with sesame seed spread (tahini)

Source: Adapted from James Braly, M.D., *Dr. Braly's Food Allergy and Nutrition Revolution.*

Why Are Amino Acids Important?

Amino acids link together to form proteins that make up muscle fiber, bone, hair, collagen, and connective tissue; that form the basis of hemoglobin, hormones, antibodies, and digestive enzymes; that assist in the transmission of nerve impulses; and that form DNA and RNA, our genetic material.

Deficiencies of amino acids can lead to viral and bacterial infections, degenerative diseases, neurologic disorders, and the breakdown of the immune system.

Essential amino acids can only be obtained from dietary sources. Nonessential amino acids can be produced from other nutrients or from the breakdown of other amino acids. A variety of quality protein is the best source of amino acids.

The need for protein is higher during the growing years of childhood. Extra protein may be necessary when nursing, when trying to overcome severe malnutrition, or when recovering from a serious illness, burn, injury, or surgery. The normal healthy adult requires only two to four ounces of quality protein per day. Most Americans eat more than four ounces of protein per meal! Remember: Excessive protein ingestion can put extra stress on the kidneys and liver and can also contribute to loss of calcium through the urine, thereby weakening your bones.

Amino Acid	Functions of Amino Acids
Arginine and ornithine	• Stimulates the release of human growth hormone (HGH). • HGH enhances immune system, strengthens bones, and connective tissue, prevents abnormal blood clotting, and increases muscle strength.
D-, L-Phenylalanine	• Builds protein tissue. • May reduce appetite. • Acts as a brain neurotransmitter. • Aids in release of endorphins to relieve pain.
L-Carnitine	• Improves fat metabolism. • Lowers cholesterol. • Transports fatty acids. • Improves cardiac function.
L-Glutamine	• Fuels metabolism. • Necessary for treatment of alcoholism. • Prevents muscle breakdown. • Maintains lining of gastrointestinal tract.
L-Lysine	• Assists formation of collagen. • Aids in repair of bones, connective tissue, and cartilage. • Necessary for production of antibodies, hormones, and enzymes. • May be useful in treating herpes virus. • May prevent gallstones.

Amino Acid	Functions of Amino Acids
L-Taurine	• Affects nerve conduction and hypersensitivity. • Vital for solubility of bile. • Balances sodium and potassium in heart muscle. • May lower triglyceride levels.
L-Tryptophan	• Converted to serotonin, which regulates nerve impulses and sleep. • Decreases incidence of migraine headaches. • Essential in production of niacin. • Assists metabolism of essential fatty acids. • Helpful in relaxation and depression.

Why Are Enzymes Important?

Enzymes are frequently proteins which facilitate biochemical reactions and are a necessary part of metabolic pathways. They play a vital role in the digestion and assimilation of foods and are essential for the absorption of vitamins and minerals.

There are actually two main types of enzymes: digestive enzymes and metabolic enzymes. The digestive enzymes are secreted by the gastrointestinal tract in an effort to help break down foods. They enable our nutrients to get absorbed more efficiently. The three main digestive enzymes include amylase, lipase, and protease, and all three are secreted by the pancreas and intestinal tract. Amylase assists the breakdown of carbohydrates, while lipase helps fat digestion, and protease aids in protein digestion.

Metabolic enzymes, on the other hand, help to assist natually occurring chemical reactions in our cells. They help to produce energy and assist in the detoxification pathways in the liver and intestinal tract. Metabolic enzymes are found in all cells and tissues and are an essential part of keeping us well. An example of one of the more important metabolic enzymes is superoxide dismutase (SOD), an antioxidant that protects our cells from free radicals. Another enzyme, catalase, helps to break down naturally occurring hydrogen peroxide, a cellular metabolic waste product, so that your body can utilize oxygen more efficiently.

Many foods are also rich sources of enzymes. These include sprouts, avocados, bananas, mangoes, papaya, and pineapple. Interestingly, pineapple is well known for its anti-inflammatory enzyme, bromelain, which can be used to help heal sport injuries or sprains more rapidly.

Coenzyme Q_{10} (CoQ_{10}) is another example of an important enzyme. CoQ_{10} is a nontoxic, fat-soluble, antioxidant nutrient, manufactured within our bodies. It plays a vital role in the production of adenosine triphosphate (ATP), the basic energy molecule of all cells. Because CoQ_{10} levels decline with age and illness, a CoQ_{10} deficiency may be a contributing factor to degenerative disease. Furthermore, CoQ_{10} is also depleted by cholesterol-lowering "statin" drugs. I always supplement my patients with extra CoQ_{10} if they are taking these medications.

WHAT ARE THE BENEFITS OF CoQ_{10}?

- Reduces hypertension.
- Slows the aging process.
- Aids in liver disease.
- Reduces periodontal disease.
- Stimulates immune system.
- Alleviates angina pain.
- Strengthens heart muscle.
- Improves chronic fatigue syndrome (CFS).
- Reduces symptoms of congestive heart failure.
- Improves exercise tolerance.

What Is Glutathione?

Glutathione is a potent antioxidant, essential for maintaining good health. It is a naturally occurring substance found in fresh fruits and vegetables. Glutathione (GSH) is composed of three essential amino acids: cysteine, glutamic acid, and glycine. Glutathione is felt to be an important enzyme to protect against the hazardous effects of free radicals. It has been shown to enhance immune response, assist in liver detoxification, prevent and treat environmental illnesses, and protect against cancer. It may also play a role in autoimmune diseases and heart disease and may protect your eyes against cataracts and macular degeneration. Statistically, people with AIDS have lower glutathione levels than individuals without this disease. I have recommended supplements of glutathione on numerous occasions to patients with liver congestion, hepatitis, chronic infections, or chemical sensitivities.

Glutathione is found in higher quanitities in raw or steamed fruits and vegetables than those that are cooked at high temperatures for long periods of time. Some of the vegetables you should consider to boost your glutathione level include acorn squash, asparagus, avocado, potatoes, and fruits such as grapefruit, strawberries, and watermelon. Lean meats, whole grains, and wheat germ are also good sources for glutathione. Some foods such as eggs, cabbage, Brussels sprouts, and kale contain substances that may help your body to natually produce more glutathione on its own. Unfortunately, glutathione levels appear to decline as you get older, making you more susceptible to the diseases of aging. Maintaining a diet rich in fresh fruits and vegetables is once again vitally important.

CHAPTER 3

Carbohydrates and Sugars

All sugars, both simple such as those found in white bread, and complex which can be found in brown rice, are converted to glycogen and ultimately stored as fat if they are not burned as energy. Although simple sugars should be minimized in your diet, complex carbohydrates which include fruits, vegetables, beans, and grains, should make up the majority of your total caloric intake.

What's the Difference between Simple and Complex Sugars?

Simple Sugars

Foods containing simple sugars cause the pancreas to release insulin rapidly. Simple sugars are not stored in the body. They are metabolized quickly, using up all of their energy instantly.

Major Sources
- *Glucose (grape sugar)**
- *Fructose (fruit sugar)**
- *Dextrose (corn sugar)**
- *Sucrose (cane and beet sugar)**
- *Molasses*
- *Maple sugar*
- *Honey*
- *White flour*
- *White rice*

* When these foods are commercially processed, simple sugars are formed.

Complex Sugars

Foods containing complex sugars take longer to break down. They are excellent sources of energy. Unlike simple carbohydrates, complex carbohydrates are stored in the body and can be converted to sugar for energy when needed. This avoids the highs and lows one experiences when eating simple sugars.

Major Sources
- *Whole fruits*
- *Vegetables*
- *Whole grains*
- *Whole-grain cereals*
- *Whole-grain breads*
- *Legumes*

Note: When whole fruit is converted to a juice, the remaining juice may act more like a simple sugar.

WHAT ARE THE BEST SOURCES OF COMPLEX CARBOHYDRATES?

	Serving Size	Carbohydrates (g)	% Calories from Carbohydrates
Apple	1 small	16	100
Blueberries	1 cup	20	100
Peaches	2 small	20	100
Apricots	3	12	96
Parsnips	⅔ cup cooked	20	96
Winter squash	¾ cup	14	96
Pumpkin, fresh	1 cup cooked	9	95
Potato, baked	2 ½ oz	18	94
Pumpkin, canned	1 cup	15	94
Sweet potatoes	⅓ cup cooked	21	94
Barley	⅓ cup cooked	16	91
Snap beans	1 cup cooked	10	89
Brown rice	⅓ cup cooked	13	88
Cornmeal	½ cup cooked	18	87
Kasha (buckwheat)	⅓ cup cooked	18	87
Bulgur	⅓ cup cooked	14	85
Corn kernels	½ cup	17	85
Spaghetti, enriched	½ cup cooked	20	84
Brussels sprouts	1 cup cooked	13	80
Corn tortilla	1	13	80
Popcorn, air popped	3 cups	18	80
Bagel	half	19	76
Black-eyed peas	⅓ cup cooked	12	76
Peas	½ cup cooked	12	76
Black beans	⅓ cup cooked	14	75
Great Northern beans	⅓ cup cooked	13	74
Rye bread	1 slice	12	74
Kidney beans	⅓ cup cooked	14	73
Oatmeal	½ cup	13	72
Lentils	⅓ cup cooked	13	72
Wheatena	½ cup cooked	14	71

Why Should We Limit Our Intake of Processed or Refined Sugar?

Processed or refined sugar comprises approximately one-eighth of our total diet. There is growing evidence that sugar can be a contributing factor in diabetes, hypoglycemia, high blood pressure, cardiac irregularities, headaches, arteriosclerosis, hyperactivity, hyperinsulinism, colitis, dental cavities, obesity, depletion of nutrients (especially B vitamins, magnesium, chromium, and manganese), and elevated cholesterol, triglycerides, and uric acid levels. If that's not enough, ingesting sugar inhibits the germ-fighting abilities of white cells for up to four hours after consumption, thereby increasing susceptibility to infection. Refined sugar provides only empty calories, devoid of nutritional value.

A good deal of refined or processed sugar is "hidden" in foods that are baked, prepackaged, canned, or frozen. Read labels to see if the total amount of sugar you are getting is higher than you think. Check to see how much sugar you and your family eat for breakfast!

How Much Sugar Is in Your Breakfast Cereal?

SUGAR CONTENT OF READY-TO-EAT CEREALS

Product	Calories per Serving	Grams of Sugar	% Sugar per Serving
All-Bran	80	6	30
Alpha-Bits, Frosted	130	13	40
Alpha Bits, Marshmallow	120	14	47
Apple Jacks	120	16	53
Basic 4	200	14	28
Bran Flakes	100	6	24
Cap'n Crunch	110	12	44
Cap'n Crunch, All Berries	130	15	46
Cap'n Crunch, Crunch Berries	100	12	48
Cap'n Crunch, Peanut Butter Crunch	110	9	33
Cheerios	110	3	11
Cheerios, Apple Cinnamon	120	13	43
Cheerios, Frosted	120	13	43
Cheerios, Honey Nut	120	11	37
Cheerios, MultiGrain Plus	110	6	22
Cinnamon Toast Crunch	130	10	31
Cocoa Krispies	120	14	47
Cocoa Pebbles	120	13	43
Cocoa Puffs	120	14	47
Cookie Crisp	120	12	40
Corn Chex	110	3	11
Corn Flakes	100	2	8
Corn Pops	120	14	47

Product	Calories per Serving	Grams of Sugar	% Sugar per Serving
Cracklin' Oat Bran	190	15	82
Crispix	110	3	11
Fiber One	60	0	0
French Toast Crunch	120	12	40
Frosted Flakes	120	14	47
Froot Loops	120	15	50
Fruity Pebbles	110	12	44
Golden Grahams	120	10	8
Grape Nuts	200	7	14
Grape Nuts Flakes	100	5	20
Healthy Choice Brown Sugar	190	9	19
Healthy Choice Mueslix	200	17	34
Healthy Choice Raisin, Almond	210	12	23
Honey Bunches of Oats, Almond	130	6	18
Honey Bunches of Oats, Honey Roasted	120	6	20
Honeycomb	110	11	40
Honey Nut Chex	120	9	3
Just Right	220	15	27
Kix	120	12	10
Life	120	6	20
Lucky Charms	120	13	43
MiniWheats, Frosted	180	10	22
Multi Bran Chex	200	12	24
Oatmeal Crisp, Almond	220	16	29
Oatmeal Crisp, Raisin	210	19	36
100% Bran	80	7	35
Oreo O's	110	11	40
Product 19	100	4	16
Puffed Rice	50	0	0
Puffed Wheat	50	0	0
Raisin Bran, Kellogg's	200	18	36
Raisin Bran, Post	190	20	42
Rice Chex	120	2	6
Rice Krispies, Razzle Dazzle	110	10	36
Smacks	100	15	60
Smart Start	180	15	33
Special K	110	4	15
Toasted Oatmeal	190	11	23
Total Corn Flakes	110	3	11
Total Raisin Bran	180	19	42
Total Whole Grain	110	5	18
Trix	120	13	43
Wheat Chex	180	5	11
Wheaties	110	4	15

Try to eat cereals that contain less than 20 percent sugar per serving. It would be even more ideal to choose those that are less than 10 percent. Since some breakfast cereals are made with refined flours and loaded with sugars, look for brands made with high-quality, unrefined grains, devoid of preservatives and artificial coloring agents, and low in refined sugars. Recommended brands include Arrowhead Mills, Barbara's, Health Valley, Lifestream, and Nature's Path.

What Is the Per Capita Consumption of Sugar in the United States?

Look at the escalation of our sugar consumption over the years! In the early 1800s, when the process of refining sugar became more efficient, the per capita consumption of sugar soared. Sugar consumption during the last 150 years has continued to rise from approximately 14 pounds per person per year in 1840 to 123 pounds per person per year in 1983 to over 135 pounds per person per year today.

What Are the Sources of Your Sugar Intake?

The following pie graph illustrates the distribution of sugar in the typical American diet. Note that many soft drinks contain a high sugar content and account for a quarter of all sugar consumption.

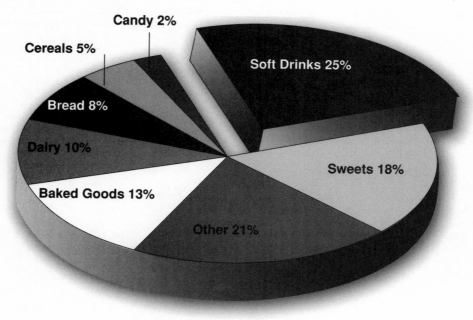

How Much Processed Sugar Is in Your Favorite Beverage?

Everyday beverages are often loaded with hidden sugar. Check the table below for the approximate sugar content in various beverages. While individual products vary in their exact calories, these numbers serve as a general guideline.

SUGAR CONTENT OF COMMON BEVERAGES

Beverage	Serving Size	Sugar Calories (% of Total Calories)	Teaspoons of Sugar per Serving
Liqueurs, cordials	.7 oz	33	1.5
Brandy, cognac	1.0 oz	41	1.7
Dessert wine	3.5 oz	35	3.0
Chocolate instant breakfast drinks	1 packet	33–37	2.3–3.0
Chocolate-flavored drinks	3–4 tsp	77–91	3.8–4.5
Iced tea, sugar-sweetened	9.0 oz	97–100	3.5–5.7
Hot cocoa mix	1.0 oz	84	5.8
Powdered drink mixes	8.0 oz	100	6.0
Cranberry juice cocktail	8.0 oz	73	6.4
Canned fruit drinks	8.0 oz	89–100	6.5–7.6
Ginger ale	12.0 oz	95	8.0
Tonic water	12.0 oz	98	8.4
Carbonated beverages	12.0 oz	95–100	8.0–11.8

What Are Your Alternatives to Table Sugar?

Fortunately, there are a variety of alternatives to plain table sugar. The table below will allow you to make more informed decisions when choosing options to sugar.

Sugar Source	Where to Find It
Barley malt syrup	Produced in a complicated process by heating sprouted barley grains in brewing vats; metabolizes slower than simple sugar; contains minimal amounts of minerals and some B vitamins.
Brown sugar	Made by adding a little molasses to white sugar; nutritionally equivalent to white sugar; 91–96% sucrose.
Corn syrup	Moderately sweet product formed when corn starch is partially broken down with acids; per capita production is 48 pounds per year; can be addictive and provoke allergic responses.
Corn sweetener	Made from corn starch; dextrose, glucose, maltose, and corn syrup are derivatives.
Dextrose	Hundreds of dextrose molecules linked end to end make up starch molecules.
Fructose	One of several sugars found in fruit; raises blood sugar levels less than dextrose and sucrose; less of a problem for diabetics.
High-fructose corn syrup	Derived from corn; may contain anywhere from 42–90% fructose; most of the rest is dextrose; is inexpensive and rapidly replacing sucrose.
Honey	Processed honey is sweeter, stickier, and much more expensive; nutritionally equivalent to table sugar; raises blood sugar levels more than sucrose; unprocessed raw honey may have more nutritional value.
Lactose	The sugar naturally found in milk and other dairy products; less sweet than table sugar.
Malt syrup	Made from sprouted grains.
Maltodextrin	Processed from corn; found in dehydrated products.
Mannitol	Found in seaweed and plants; body cannot digest; can cause diarrhea and kidney problems.
Maple syrup	Processed from maple tree sap; 60–75% sucrose.
Molasses	Thick, dark syrup formed in the production of sucrose from sugar cane; molasses, especially blackstrap molasses, contains significant amounts of minerals such as iron, calcium, and phosphorus.
Raw sugar	Produced when sugar cane juice is evaporated; retains minimal nutrients found in raw cane sugar; not particularly nutritious.
Rice syrup	Metabolizes more slowly than sucrose; contains fewer nutrients than barley malt syrup but more B vitamins and minerals than honey.
Sorbitol	Commercial sorbitol is made from dextrose; in natural forms, primarily found in berries, apples, pears, cherries, plums, seaweed, and algae.

Sugar Source	Where to Find It
Sorghum	Production process similar to molasses; rich in minerals such as calcium, iron, and potassium, as well as B vitamins.
Stevia	Derived from the leaves of the stevia plant; contains no calories; does not affect blood glucose levels; excellent sweetener for diabetics and hypoglycemics; lowers elevated blood pressure without affecting normal blood pressure; inhibits the growth and reproduction of bacteria that cause tooth decay and gum disease.
Sucanat	Derived from fresh sugar cane juice; evaporated so that vitamins and minerals remain.
Sucrose	Ordinary table sugar; made from sugar cane and sugar beets. Each sucrose molecule is composed of one fructose molecule and one dextrose molecule; contains no nutritional value.
Turbinado	Produced when molasses and impurities are removed from raw sugar; without nutrient-rich molasses, it contains more empty calories than raw sugar.
Xylitol	Made from xylos, a wood sugar, and corn cobs, peanut shells, coconut shells, wheat straw, and cotton seed hulls; causes diarrhea; banned abroad.

What Are the Most Desirable Natural Sweeteners?

If you continually sweeten your foods, try to substitute with more natural and healthier sweetening agents whenever possible. In general, using sources of fruit is a good option in place of table sugar. I also suggest limiting your intake of artificial sweeteners since it's always advantageous to go with more natural wholesome foods.

There have been two new low-calorie sweetening agents that are making their way onto the grocery store shelves. Sucralose is a low-calorie sweetener that is made by chemically altering sugar. It is thought to be 600 times sweeter than sugar, does not contain any calories, and passes through the body unchanged. Since it is highly stable under a variety of processing conditions, it can be used wherever sugar is used; for example, during cooking or baking.

A second calorie-free sweetener known as Acesulfame-K, or Acesulfame potassium, is actually 200 times sweeter than Sucralose. Even though this substance was approved in 1988 as a tabletop sweetener, it was recently approved for use in soft drinks as well. It is excreted through the gastrointestinal tract unchanged and is therefore noncaloric. Acesulfame-K is now being combined with Aspartame in some soft drinks since the combination is sweeter than either sweetener used alone.

A third calorie-free natural sweetener, stevia, grows wild as a tropical herb in Paraguay and Brazil. It is the most popular sugar substitute used in Japan and can be found in gum, yogurt, and soft drinks. Stevia is 100 to 200 times sweeter than table sugar and has a slightly bitter aftertaste. Because it is so sweet, only small amounts are needed. As it does not break down in heat, it can be used in your tea or coffee. In general, all of the natural sweeteners below are more desirable than plain table sugar. However, some may be more desirable than others.

NATURAL SWEETENERS

More Desirable

The following whole foods can be safely used as sweeteners, unless you are unable to tolerate them:

• Dates
• Dried fruits, such as raisins and apricots
• Fruit purees
• Fruit juice
• Fruit conserve

Less Desirable

If you feel you must use added sweeteners, it is preferable to use those that are less refined and retain more of their nutrients. The "natural" sweeteners below contain sugars that can affect blood sugar levels in the same way that white sugar can. The body converts them to glucose at varying rates. You may want to experiment with different sweetening agents to see which ones you can best tolerate.

• Raw honey
• Unsulphured blackstrap molasses
• Fig concentrate
• Rice syrup
• Sucanat
• Stevia
• Carob powder
• Natural maple syrup (without corn syrup added)

ARTIFICIAL SWEETENERS

The artificial sweetener, aspartame, marketed as Equal® or NutriSweet®, is composed of three ingredients: the amino acids phenylalanine, aspartic acid, and methyl alcohol. Although aspartame is FDA approved and is used in thousands of food products, it remains a controversial substance in our food supply. In my practice, I have noted that aspartame can aggravate a variety of symptoms ranging from headaches to blurred vision and mental confusion to neurologic impairment. Because aspartame can break down when heated, do not cook with it. Aspartame, as well as other artificial sweeteners such as saccharin and cyclamate, has been linked to cancer. For these reasons, try to avoid all products containing aspartame.

Could Your Headaches or Depression Be Due to Diet Soda?

Aspartame has been associated with a variety of symptoms including:

- Headaches
- Dizziness
- Seizures
- Nausea
- Numbness
- Muscle spasm

- Fatigue
- Blurred vision
- Irritability
- Heart palpitations
- Memory lapse
- Insomnia

Aspartame has been associated with a wide range of diseases including:

- Birth defects
- Brain tumors
- Chronic fatigue syndrome

- Diabetes
- Epilepsy
- Fibromyalgia

Where are artificial sweeteners found?

Artificial sugars are found in over 7,000 products including:

- Soft drinks
- Iced tea
- Drink mixes
- Candy
- Gelatin desserts

- Chewing gum
- Children's vitamins
- Children's medications
- Diabetic products
- Most diet products

CHAPTER 4

Fats, Oils, and Essential Fatty Acids

Fats are lipids that are solid at room temperature, whereas oils are fats that are liquid at room temperature. We can either ingest fats from our foods or manufacture them from excessive carbohydrate intake. One gram of fat contains twice as many calories as one gram of protein or carbohydrate. Because there has been much negative press regarding the intake of fats, let's take a look at some of the real issues at stake here.

Why Are Fats Important?

Fats are an important source of energy and are an integral constituent of all cell membranes. They help to regulate body temperature and conserve body heat.

Interestingly enough, the majority of our brain and liver is composed of fat. Fats are required for the absorption of fat-soluble vitamins: A, D, E, and K. Although fats certainly have some negative health effects, they are necessary for the formation of hormones such as estrogen, progesterone, and testosterone. Therefore, fat intake should not be severely restricted.

However, ingesting excessive quantities of fat has been linked to heart disease, vascular disease, cancer, obesity, and diabetes. It is crucial to limit the amount of total fat in our diets, especially saturated fat and unnatural partially hydrogenated fats.

All fats are a mix of saturated, monounsaturated, and polyunsaturated fatty acids, but the proportions vary greatly. Since saturated fat has the most detrimental effect on the body, try to select foods low in saturated fat and higher in monounsaturated and polyunsaturated fat.

For example, avocados have a higher percentage of calories from fat than pot roast, but the fat content is predominantly monounsaturated. In contrast, pot roast is lower in the percentage of calories from fat, but higher in unhealthy saturated fat. Strive to reduce or ultimately eliminate partially hydrogenated fat from your diet completely. These partially hydrogenated fats are commonly found in baked products such as crackers, doughnuts, cakes, and pies. I will be discussing this in more detail on page 50.

How Much Fat Should You Ingest Each Day?

Ideally, fat intake should be limited to no more than 25 percent of your total daily caloric intake. For example, if you strive to maintain a diet consisting of 1,500 calories per day and consume no more than 20 percent of your calories from fat, be sure to limit your fat intake to no more than 33 grams of fat per day. Check labels and the table in the Cholesterol section on pages 57–63, for information regarding the number of grams of fat per serving. Since saturated fat has been linked to chronic degenerative diseases, it is advisable to limit your saturated fat intake to less than one-third of your total fat intake. Therefore, polyunsaturated and monounsaturated fat should comprise two-thirds of your total fat intake.

GUIDELINES FOR DAILY FAT INTAKE

If you are trying to maintain a diet of no more than 1,500 calories per day and at the same time eat no more than 20 percent of your calories from fat, consume no more than 33 grams of fat each day. Since you may find that it is more efficient for you simply to count the number of grams of fat each day, the following table indicates the upper limits for the number of grams of fat if you are trying to maintain a 1,500-, 2,000-, or a 2,500-calorie diet per day.

Daily Calories	30% Fat (g)	20% Fat (g)	10% Fat (g)
1,500	50	33	16
2,000	67	44	22
2,500	83	56	28

Where Is Fat Found?

The following table lists the percentage of fat calories in some common items.

Sources of Dietary Fat	Total*	Saturated Fat (g)	Monounsaturated Fat (g)	Polyunsaturated Fat (g)	% Calories from Fat (g)
Coconut oil (1 tbsp)	14	111.8	0.8	0.2	100
Corn oil (1 tbsp)	14	1.7	3.3	8.0	100
Olive oil (1 tbsp)	14	1.8	9.9	1.1	100
Palm kernel oil (1 tbsp)	14	11.1	1.5	0.2	100
Butter (1 tbsp)	11	7.1	3.3	0.4	99
Avocado (half)	15	2.3	9.7	1.7	89
Walnuts (1 oz)	16	1.0	3.36	10.6	85
Peanuts, dry-roasted (1 oz)	15	2.0	8.9	3.1	79
Cheddar cheese (1 oz)	9	6	2.7	0.3	70
Egg (whole)	6	1.7	2.2	0.7	66
Whole milk (1 cup)	8	5.1	2.4	0.3	48
Pot roast (trimmed 3½ oz)	13	5	6	0.5	45
Ham (trimmed 3½ oz)	11	3.8	5	1.4	45
Salmon (3½ oz)	11	2	5	2	45
Top round (3½ oz)	6	2.3	2.5	0.3	28
Chicken, light meat (without skin, 3½ oz)	4	1	1.3	0.3	20
Turkey, light meat (without skin, 3½ oz)	3	0.9	0.5	0.7	18
Whole wheat bread (1 slice)	1	0.4	0.4	0.3	14
Oatmeal (½ cup)	1	0.2	0.4	0.5	12
Cantaloupe (⅓)	0.6	0.06	0.06	0.2	9
Black beans (⅓ cup)	0.3	0.03	0.03	0.2	4
Brown rice (⅓ cup)	0.3	0.1	0.1	0.1	4
Lentils (⅓ cup)	0.3	0.03	0.03	0.2	4
Nonfat milk (1 cup)	0.4	0.3	0.1	trace	4
Asparagus (1 cup cooked)	1	0.1	trace	0.2	2
Egg white	0	0	0	0	0
Carrot (1 raw)	0	0	0	0	0
Grapefruit (half)	0	0	0	0	0

* Figures for saturated, monounsaturated, and polyunsaturated fats may not add up to the total fat amount because this measurement includes other fat components such as triglycerides, plant sterols, glycerols, and fat-soluble vitamins present in foods.

Source: Since the author is unknown, we are reprinting this in good faith.

How Can I Choose Low-Fat Foods?

The following table illustrates the percentage of fat calories in various foods. A sirloin steak is 83 percent fat, while a grapefruit is 2 percent fat! Use this table as a reference when selecting low-fat foods.

PERCENTAGES OF CALORIES FROM FAT

Meats

Sirloin steak	83
Pork sausage	83
T-bone steak	82
Porterhouse steak	82
Bacon, lean	82
Rib roast	81
Bologna	81
Sausage	81
Spareribs	80
Hot dogs	80
Lamb rib chops	79
Duck meat, with skin	76
Salami	76
Liverwurst	75
Rump roast	71
Ham	69
Stewing beef	66
Goose meat, with skin	65
Ground beef, lean	64
Veal breast	64
Leg of lamb	61
Chicken, dark meat, with skin	56
Round steak	53
Chuck rib roast	50
Chuck steak	50
Turkey, dark meat, with skin	47
Lamb chops, lean	45
Chicken, light meat, with skin	44

Vegetables

Mustard greens	13
Kale	13
Beet greens	12
Lettuce	12
Turnip greens	11
Mushrooms	8
Cabbage	7
Cauliflower	7
Eggplant	7
Asparagus	6
Green beans	6
Celery	6
Cucumber	6
Turnip	6
Zucchini	6
Carrots	4
Green peas	4
Artichokes	3
Onions	3
Beets	2
Potatoes	1

Grains

Oatmeal	16
Buckwheat, dark	7
Rye, dark	7
Whole wheat	5
Brown rice	5
Corn flour	5
Bulgur	4
Barley	3
Buckwheat, light	3
Rye, light	2
Wild rice	2

Fish

Tuna, oil-packed	63
Herring	59
Anchovies	54
Sea bass	53
Perch	53
Caviar, Sturgeon	52
Mackerel	50
Sardines, in oil	49
Salmon	49

Nuts and Seeds

Coconut	85
Walnuts	79
Sesame seeds	76
Almonds	76
Sunflower seeds	71
Pumpkin seeds	71
Cashews	70
Peanuts	69
Chestnuts	7

Legumes

Tofu	49
Soybeans	37
Soybean sprouts	28
Garbanzo beans	11
Kidney beans	4
Lima beans	4
Mung bean sprouts	4
Lentils	3
Broad beans	3
Mung beans	3

Fruits

Olive	91
Avocado	82
Grape	11
Strawberry	11
Apple	8
Blueberry	7
Lemon	7
Pear	5
Apricot	4
Orange	4
Cherry	4
Banana	4
Cantaloupe	3
Pineapple	3
Grapefruit	2
Papaya	2
Peach	2
Prune	1

Dairy Products

Butter	100
Cream, whipping	92
Cream cheese	90
Cream, light	85
Egg yolks	85
Half and Half	79
Blue cheese	73
Cheddar cheese	71
Swiss cheese	68
Ricotta cheese, whole milk	66
Eggs, whole	65
Mozzarella cheese, part skim	55
Goat's milk	54
Cow's milk	49
Yogurt, plain	49
Cottage cheese	35
Milk, low fat (2%)	31
Yogurt, low fat	31
Ice milk	29
Cottage cheese, nonfat	21

What Are Trans-Fatty Acids?

Trans-fatty acids are produced by the process of partially hydrogenating vegetable oils. They are often found in processed foods, including pastries, cookies, crackers, and margarines. They were introduced into human foods in 1910.

Hydrogenation is a chemical process that occurs when hydrogen molecules are added to monounsaturated or polyunsaturated fatty acids, thereby making them more saturated. Hydrogenation is used to convert a liquid oil to a semisolid or solid state at room temperature. For example, vegetable oils are often partially hydrogenated to produce shortening or margarines. The hydrogenation process increases the stability of a fat or oil, which is important in cooking or extending a product's shelf life. All fats and polyunsaturated fats in particular are susceptible to breaking down when exposed to air, heat, or sunlight. If an oil becomes oxidized, it may impart a rancid flavor or odor. The degree of hydrogenation of a particular food can also influence its characteristics. For example, hydrogenation can affect the spreadability of margarine, the flakiness of pie crust, or the creaminess of puddings. Oils can be hydrogenated to a lesser or greater extent, depending on the desired use for the food. In either case, hydrogen molecules are added to the oil. Generally speaking, most packaged foods will list whether or not partially hydrogenated vegetable oils are contained in that particular product. Because hydrogenated vegetable oils have been shown to have adverse health effects, intake should be severely restricted.

Adverse effects of consuming trans-fatty acids include the following:

- Lowers HDL ("good") cholesterol.
- Raises LDL ("bad") cholesterol.
- Raises total cholesterol levels.
- Is associated with low infant birthweight.
- Has adverse effect on immune system.
- Increases risk of diabetes.
- Potentiates free radical formation.
- Lowers milk quality of lactating females.

During hydrogenation, an abnormal fat is formed whereby the hydrogen atom moves to the opposite side of a double bond. This then forms a trans-fat, which has been associated with a wide range of adverse health effects, as listed above.

Since fats are certainly an integral part of health and normal metabolism, you should strive to cautiously select the appropriate foods that are either low in fat or rich in essential fatty acids. The pages in this chapter will help you to make prudent dietary choices.

In general, most plant-derived foods such as fruit, vegetables, grains, beans, and legumes are lower in fat content than animal-derived foods such as beef, pork, chicken, turkey, and lamb. Furthermore, plant-based foods contain no cholesterol at all as cholesterol is only found in animal-derived foods. For these reasons, most people find that eating wholesome foods in a near vegetarian diet is a healthy way of eating. Adding fish such as salmon, cod, tuna, halibut, and sea bass to your diet is also suggested since these fish are high in the beneficial essential fatty acids.

Margarine Versus Butter

While you may have been led to believe that margarine is preferable to butter, margarine is far from perfect. Since it contains high amounts of partially hydrogenated oils, it may actually raise your LDL cholesterol and lower the beneficial HDL cholesterol. On the other hand, butter is composed of 100 percent saturated fats, which should also be limited. For these reasons, I would suggest leaning toward olive or canola oil, which contain higher amounts of monounsaturated fats, while limiting your intake of both margarine and butter.

Do I Have to Give Up Cheese?

Cheese is an extremely high-fat food. If you are watching your fat intake, you should make an effort to select low-fat cheeses. The following table lists various cheeses and their percentage of fat.

PERCENTAGES OF CALORIES FROM FAT IN VARIOUS CHEESES

90	Cream cheese	68	Mozzarella, regular
81	Roquefort, blue cheese	67	Ricotta, whole milk
78	Feta	66	Swiss cheese or Provolone
75	American cheese	59	Parmesan
74	Cheddar	56	Mozzarella, part skim
74	Brie	52	Ricotta, part skim
70	Muenster	25–50	"Light" or "diet" cheeses

How Can You Calculate Fat Grams?

Use the following formula to calculate the percentage of fat calories in the food you eat:

---

1 gram of fat = 9 calories
If a serving has 5 grams of fat, then:
5 x 9 = 45 calories from fat

If the total calories of a serving are 100, then:
45 divided by 100 = 45% of calories from fat

One gram of protein or carbohydrates equals only four calories. Therefore, you can eat almost twice the quantity of protein or carbohydrates as compared to fats and still be eating the same number of calories!

FAT DEFINITIONS USED BY THE FDA

Low fat = *less than 3 grams of fat per serving*

Low saturated fat = *less than 1 gram per serving, 15% of calories from saturated fat*

Fat free = *less than ¹/₂ gram fat or saturated fat per serving*

Reduced fat = *at least 25% less fat than usual for that product*

Light = *¹/₂ the fat or ¹/₂ the calories of its regular counterpart*

Lean = *less than 10 grams of fat, 4 grams of saturated fat, and 95 milligrams of cholesterol per serving*

Cholesterol free = *less than 2 milligrams of cholesterol and 2 grams of saturated fat per serving*

TIPS

The labeling of milk can be very confusing. This should make it simpler.

- 2% milk is labeled reduced-fat milk.
- 2% milk is not low in fat.
- 2% milk contains 120 calories, 5 grams of fat, and 3 grams of saturated fat per cup.
- 1% milk contains 100 calories, 2.5 grams of fat, and 1.5 grams of saturated fat per cup.
- Skim milk contains 80 calories and 0 fat per cup.
- Whole milk contains 150 calories, 8 grams of fat, and 5 grams of saturated fat per cup.
- Switching from whole milk to skim milk can greatly reduce your intake of saturated fat. If you drink 7 ounces of skim milk per day instead of whole milk after the age of two, you could save 1.5 million calories over the course of a lifetime, which is enough to put on 400 pounds!

What Are the Three Major Types of Fats Found in Oils?

Monounsaturated

Lowers the "bad" LDL cholesterol without lowering the "good" HDL cholesterol.
Limit intake to 10–15 percent of total daily calories.

Polyunsaturated

Reduces both "bad" LDL and "good" HDL cholesterol.
Limit intake to 5–10 percent of total daily calories.

Saturated

Raises serum cholesterol and contributes to heart disease.
Limit intake to less than 10 percent of daily calories.

Which Oils Should I Select?

Strive to select polyunsaturated and monounsaturated fats and oils. Limit oils that are high in saturated fats.

Use

Avocado oil	Mostly monounsaturated; puree and use instead of butter or margarine.
Almond oil	High in monounsaturated fat.
Canola oil	Greatly monounsaturated, less fat than any other oil; use for general purposes.
Fish oil	High in polyunsaturated oil and omega-3 fatty acids.
Flaxseed oil	High in polyunsaturated oil and omega-3 fatty acids.
Olive oil	More monounsaturated fat than any other oil; use only extra virgin olive oil in hot or cold dishes.
Sesame, roasted (dark)	Use in salad dressings and marinades, soups; stir-fries; highly flavorful.

Use Moderately

Sunflower, corn, sesame oils	Too high in saturated fat; use only in cold dishes.
Nut oils (walnut, hazelnut)	Polyunsaturated; use moderately in salads and cold dishes.
Soy	Mostly polyunsaturated.
Peanut	Good percentage of monounsaturates but has more saturated fat than canola oil and more polyunsaturates than olive oil.
Cocoa butter	Found in chocolate, appears saturated but not as risky.

Avoid

Butter	Very heavily saturated.
Chicken fat, lard, beef fat	Too saturated, contains cholesterol.
Cottonseed oil	Too high in saturated fat, too low in monounsaturated fat.
Margarine	Heavily hydrogenated.
Palm, palm kernel, and coconut oils	Too high in saturated fat.
Safflower oil	Too saturated.
Vegetable shortening	Oils have been deformed by chemical processing.

How Much Saturated Fat Is in the Butter You Use?

All fats are a mixture of saturated, monounsaturated, and polyunsaturated fatty acids. However, their proportions vary greatly. For example, olive oil has more healthful monounsaturates than any other oils. On the other hand, animal products such as butter and lard, contain higher percentages of saturated fat and cholesterol. Strive to reduce your total fat calories.

Monounsaturated Fats: Diets high in monounsaturates lower "bad" LDL cholesterol without lowering "good" HDL. Keep monounsaturates between 10 and 15 percent of total daily calories.

Oil	% Mono	% Poly	% Sat	Comments
Olive	77	9	14	Olive oil appears to have the cholesterol-lowering benefits of polyunsaturates without the drawbacks. It also may help control blood pressure and diabetes.
Avocado	74	14	12	Avocado, almond, and apricot oils are good sources of monounsaturated fats.
Almond	73	18	9	However, their strong taste and high price make them unpopular choices.
Apricot	63	31	6	
Canola	62	31	7	Canola and peanut oils both have large percentages of monounsaturates. Moreover,
Peanut	48	34	18	the fatty acids in canola oil may have the same benefits for blood lipids and for lowering blood pressure as fish oils.
Margarine	46	33	21	Margarine and shortening contain hydrogenated oils and trans-fatty acids. They may
Shortening	45	27	28	have an adverse effect on the heart, blood lipids, and the immune system.
Sesame	42	43	15	Sesame oil is frequently used in Oriental cooking.

Polyunsaturated Fats: Polyunsaturates reduce both "bad" LDL and "good" HDL. A possible link between diets high in polyunsaturated fats and cancer is under investigation. Keep polyunsaturates between 5 and 10 percent of total daily calories.

Oil	% Mono	% Poly	% Sat	Comments
Safflower	13	78	9	Safflower and sunflower contain immune-boosting vitamin E.
Sunflower	20	69	11	
Walnut	24	66	10	Walnut oil should not be used to fry foods for long periods of time.
Wheat germ	16	64	20	Wheat germ oil is exceptionally rich in immune-boosting vitamin E.
Corn	25	62	13	Corn oil is a good all-purpose cooking and salad oil.
Soybean	24	61	15	Soybean oil contains linoleic acid, which is converted in the body to the same fatty acids found in fish oil, so it may also have some of the same health benefits. It is also very rich in vitamin E.
Cottonseed	19	54	27	Cottonseed oil, a cotton by-product, is found in many commercially baked goods.

Saturated Fats: High intakes of saturated fats have been shown to elevate serum cholesterol and contribute to heart disease. Keep saturated fats below 10 percent of total daily calories.

Oil	% Mono	% Poly	% Sat	Comments
Coconut	6	2	92	Coconut and palm kernel oils contain lauric acid, the fatty acid that predominates in
Palm kernel	12	2	86	some tropical oils. They have been found to be linked to plaque formation.
Butter	30	4	65	Butter and palm oil contain a relatively high percentage of monounsaturates, but also
Palm	39	10	51	an excessive amount of saturated fat. Butter also contains cholesterol.

Essential Fatty Acids

Essential fatty acids (EFAs) are fats that cannot be manufactured by the body and must be supplied by the foods we ingest. They are vital components of all cell membranes. They are precursors to hormone-like compounds (prostaglandins) that are essential for our body's well-being.

Omega-6 oils (linoleic acid) and omega-3 oils (alpha-linolenic acid) are the two major types of EFAs. A proper balance between the two is necessary. They regulate inflammation, blood pressure, heart rate, vascular dilation, blood clotting, immune system response, fat metabolism, neurological function, and cholesterol levels. Deficiencies of essential fatty acids can cause eczema, autoimmune problems, depression, premenstrual syndrome (PMS), arthritis, joint stiffness, hypertension, and prostate problems. It has been noted that most Americans do not ingest adequate quantities of foods containing essential fatty acids. Both omega-3 and omega-6 oils are important factors in our diet.

Which Oils Are the Best Sources of Essential Fatty Acids?

Oil	% Omega-3	% Omega-6
Linseed	60	20
Fish oil*	30	4
Hempseed	19	62
Walnut, English	11	55
Walnut, black	7	62
Soy	8	50
Wheat germ	10	40
Chestnut	5	40
Walnut	4	67
Beechnut	3	40
Safflower	0.5	70
Poppyseed		69
Evening Primrose Oil		60
Sunflower	0.5	60
Corn	0.5	50
Pumpkin seed		51
Cottonseed	0.5	50
Sesame	0.5	40
Cashew	0.5	20
Peanut	0.5	20
Olive	0.5	10
Coconut	0.5	3

* Salmon, cod, tuna, halibut, sea bass, sardines, haddock, and mackerel are particularly high in omega-3 fatty acids.

TIP

- When selecting oils, select those oils which are higher in mono- and polyunsaturated fats.
- Use only cold-pressed expeller oils (oils which have been extracted by a continuous auger or screw rather than a petroleum solvent such as hexane).
- Use oils which have not undergone hydrogenation.
- Although 100 percent of the calories in oils are derived from fat, when using fats, we should strive to have a lower percentage of saturated fats.
- Use more low-fat or fat-free products.
- Use herbs and spices to season foods, rather than salt and oil.
- Instead of frying foods, bake, stew, boil, or broil.

CHAPTER 5

Cholesterol

If someone eats what is useful for his health, and avoids other things that may shorten his life, then he is a man of wisdom and self-control.

—Paracelsus

Cholesterol is an odorless, white, waxy fat made by the liver. It is used to produce hormones and bile salts and to build cell walls. The liver produces most of our cholesterol. An unhealthy diet, however, can elevate your total blood cholesterol level, thereby contributing to accelerated plaque formation and the clogging of arteries. This may eventually lead to heart disease, stroke, peripheral vascular disease, hypertension, and cerebral arterial disease. It is the saturated fat in food that has the greatest effect on your cholesterol level.

What Are the Main Types of Cholesterol?

LDL (Low-Density Lipoprotein):

- Is known as "bad" cholesterol.
- Is thought to result from dietary saturated fats.
- Deposits cholesterol in artery walls.
- Is associated with heart disease.

HDL (High-Density Lipoprotein):

- Is known as "good" cholesterol.
- Helps to take dietary cholesterol back to the liver where it can be processed.
- Prevents buildup of cholesterol on artery walls.

How Can You Reduce Your Cholesterol?

- Do thirty minutes of aerobic exercise three to four times per week to raise your HDL level.
- Change the fat content of your meals to low-fat, low-cholesterol, which may reduce your blood cholesterol by 10–15 percent.
- Eat unsaturated fats.
- Eat more high-fiber foods such as fruits, vegetables, beans, rice, and whole grains.
- Lose weight.

What Should Your Cholesterol Level Be?

Your cholesterol level is usually checked as part of an overall comprehensive health evaluation. Your doctor will usually check not only the total cholesterol but also the LDL and HDL cholesterol levels as well. Since high cholesterol has been associated with coronary heart disease, hypertension, and stroke, it is desirable to keep your total cholesterol below 200 mg/dl and your LDL below 130 mg/dl. Ideally, a more desirable level for total cholesterol would range from 150 to 180 and the LDL would range from 90 to 110. Due to the protective effect of your HDL cholesterol, a desirable range would be above 35 mg/dl. In essence, the higher the HDL the better.

As a physician, I also place emphasis on the total cholesterol to HDL ratio. A desirable level would be less than 4:1. The lower the cholesterol to HDL ratio, the more protective this is against the development of coronary artery disease. On the other hand, if your ratio is greater than 5:1, you are in a higher risk range.

If you are at risk, I usually suggest a cholesterol-lowering program which includes dietary changes, a comprehensive exercise program, meditation or stress reduction, weight loss, and smoking cessation, along with a regimen of nutritional supplements including vitamins, minerals, and botanicals or herbal supplements.

So, to reduce your risk of developing heart disease, increase your HDL and lower your LDL cholesterol. For every 1 percent drop in LDL, your risk of developing heart disease is reduced by 2 percent. On the other hand, for every 1 percent increase in HDL cholesterol, your risk of heart disease drops by 3–4 percent.

Currently, more than nine million Americans take prescription cholesterol-lowering drugs on a regular basis. I always suggest to my patients to try a more natural approach first since cholesterol-lowering drugs have been associated with numerous potential side effects.

The following table presents an overview of what is generally accepted to be the upper limits for total cholesterol, LDL, and HDL cholesterol levels.

CHOLESTEROL GUIDELINES

Risk	Total Cholesterol	LDL	HDL
High	Above 239 mg/dl	Above 159 mg/dl	Less than 35 mg/dl
Borderline	200–239 mg/dl	130–159 mg/dl	35–60 mg/dl
Desirable	Below 200 mg/dl	Below 130 mg/dl	Above 60 mg/dl

Which Foods Are Lower in Fat and Cholesterol?

The following table can be used to guide you in making wise food selections. If possible, strive to keep your daily cholesterol intake to less than 300 mg per day.

FAT AND CHOLESTEROL COMPARISON TABLE

Example	Item	Saturated Fat (g)	Total Fat (g)	Cholesterol (mg)
Beef	Top round, lean, broiled	2.2	6.2	84
100 grams	Ground lean, broiled medium	7.3	18.5	87
(3½ oz)	Beef prime rib, lean, broiled	14.9	35.2	86
Processed meats	Pork and beef	6.4	17.8	47
100 grams	Sausage smoked, link, beef and pork	10.6	30.3	71
(3½ oz)	Bologna, beef	11.7	28.4	56
	Frankfurter, beef	12.0	29.4	48
	Salami	12.2	34.4	79
Pork	Ham steak, extra lean	1.4	4.2	45
100 grams	Pork, center loin	4.7	13.7	111
(3½ oz)	Pork, spareribs	11.8	30.3	121
Poultry	Chicken broilers or fryers, roasted:			
100 grams	• Light meat without skin	1.3	4.5	85
(3½ oz)	• Light meat with skin	3.1	10.9	84
	• Dark meat without skin	2.7	9.7	93
	• Dark meat with skin	4.4	15.8	91
	• Chicken skin	11.4	40.7	83
Fin fish	Cod	0.1	0.7	58
100 grams	Perch	0.2	1.2	115
(3½ oz)	Snapper	0.4	1.7	47
	Rockfish	0.5	2.0	44
	Tuna	1.6	6.3	49
	Mackerel	4.2	17.8	75
Mollusks	Clam	0.2	2.0	67
100 grams	Mussel	0.9	4.5	56
(3½ oz)	Oyster	1.3	5.0	109
Crustaceans	Crab	0.2	1.8	100
100 grams	Lobster	0.1	0.6	72
(3½ oz)	Shrimp	0.3	1.1	195
Eggs				
(1 yolk = 17 grams)	Egg yolk	1.7	5.6	272
(1 white = 33 grams)	Egg white	0.0	trace	0
(1 whole = 50 grams)	Egg, whole	1.7	5.6	272

Example	Item	Saturated Fat (g)	Total Fat (g)	Cholesterol (mg)
Nuts and seeds				
100 grams	Chestnuts	0.4	2.2	0
(3½ oz)	Almonds	4.9	51.6	0
	Sunflower seeds	5.2	49.8	0
	Pecans	5.2	64.6	0
	Walnuts	5.6	61.9	0
	Pistachio nuts	6.1	48.4	0
	Peanut kernels	6.8	49.2	0
	Cashew nuts	9.2	46.4	0
	Brazil nuts	16.2	66.1	0
Fruits				
100 grams	Peaches	0.010	0.09	0
(3½ oz)	Oranges	0.015	0.12	0
	Strawberries	0.020	0.37	0
	Apples	0.058	0.36	0
Vegetables	Cooked, boiled, drained:	0.026	0.10	0
100 grams	• Potatoes	0.034	0.18	0
(3½ oz)	• Carrots	0.042	0.26	0
	• Spinach	0.043	0.28	0
	• Broccoli	0.064	0.28	0
	• Beans, green and yellow	0.064	0.31	0
	• Squash, yellow, crookneck	0.197	1.28	0
	• Corn	1.74	8.86	0
	• Florida avocado	2.60	17.34	0
	• California avocado			
Grains and legumes	Split peas, cooked, boiled	0.054	0.39	0
	Red kidney beans, cooked, boiled	0.070	0.50	0
100 grams	Oatmeal, cooked	0.190	1.00	0
(3½ oz)				
Milk and cream	Skim milk	0.3	0.4	4
1 cup	Buttermilk (0.9% fat)	1.3	2.2	9
(8 fluid oz)	Low-fat milk (1% fat)	1.6	2.6	10
	Whole milk (3.7% fat)	5.6	8.9	35
	Light cream	28.8	46.3	159
	Heavy whipping cream	54.8	88.1	326
Yogurt and sour cream	Plain yogurt, skim milk	0.3	0.4	4
1 cup	Plain yogurt, low fat (1.6%)	2.3	3.5	14
(8 fluid oz)	Plain yogurt, whole milk	4.8	7.4	29
	Sour cream	30.0	48.2	102

Example	Item	Saturated Fat (g)	Total Fat (g)	Cholesterol (mg)
Soft cheese	Cottage cheese, low fat (1% fat)	1.5	2.3	10
1 cup	Cottage cheese, creamed	6.0	9.5	31
(8 fluid oz)	Ricotta, part skim	12.1	19.5	76
	Ricotta, whole milk	18.8	29.5	116
	American processed spread	30.2	48.1	125
	Cream cheese	49.9	79.2	250
Hard cheese	Mozzarella, part skim	22.9	36.1	132
(8 oz)	Mozzarella, whole milk	29.7	49.0	177
	Provolone	38.8	60.4	157
	Swiss	40.4	62.4	209
	Blue	42.4	65.1	170
	Brick	42.7	67.4	213
	Muenster	43.4	68.1	218
	American processed	44.7	71.1	213
	Cheddar	47.9	75.1	238
Vegetable oils and	Canola oil	14.8	218.0	0
shortening	Safflower oil	19.8	218.0	0
1 cup	Sunflower oil	22.5	218.0	0
(8 fluid oz)	Corn oil	27.7	218.0	0
	Olive oil	29.2	216.0	0
	Soybean oil	31.4	218.0	0
	Margarine, regular soft tub*	32.2	182.6	0
	Margarine, stick or brick*	34.2	182.6	0
	Peanut oil	36.4	216.0	0
	Household vegetable shortening*	51.2	205.0	0
	Cottonseed oil	56.4	218.0	0
	Palm oil	107.4	218.0	0
	Coconut oil	188.5	218.0	0
	Palm kernel oil	177.4	218.0	0
Animal fats	Chicken fat	61.2	205.0	174
1 cup	Lard	80.4	205.0	195
(8 fluid oz)	Mutton fat	96.9	205.0	209
	Beef fat	102.1	205.0	223
	Butter	114.4	183.9	496

*Made with hydrogenated soybean oil and hydrogenated cottonseed oil.

Source: US Dept. of Health & Human Services, National Institute of Health.

All animal food contains cholesterol, while all plant food is devoid of cholesterol. This is why, in part, vegetarians usually have a lower cholesterol level than people who eat a high-meat diet. In general, plant-based foods are also lower in fat than animal foods including beef, pork, lamb, or chicken.

CHAPTER 6

Wholesome Foods for Wholesome Bodies

Most health problems begin in the kitchen.
—Paul White, M.D.

"You are what you eat," or so the slogan goes. The benefits of certain foods—such as organic, high-fiber sea vegetables and grains—has been repeatedly borne out in medical and nutritional studies. The more we eat of these foods, the stronger and healthier we will be

What Are the Benefits of Organic Foods?

Organic fruits and vegetables are grown without the use of herbicides and pesticides. Many people are concerned about the potential adverse health effects of pesticides, herbicides, and fungicides, and are therefore turning to organic produce. Infants and young children are especially at risk for developing adverse reactions to pesticides and related residues because they have yet to develop mature detoxification pathways and immune systems. For these reasons, you and your family should eat organically grown food whenever possible.

Organic Foods:
- Avoid the risk of ingesting and accumulating chemicals from fertilizers, soil fumigants, pesticides, and herbicides used in commercial food production.
- Avoid the risk of exposure to dyes, waxes, sprays, and dips used to retard spoilage.
- Taste better.

Why Should You Eat Organic Foods?

According to a report in the *Journal of Applied Nutrition*, organic foods are 50 to 390 percent more nutritious in terms of trace elements than conventionally grown foods.

The following table lists findings from research at Rutgers University comparing the mineral content of vegetables that have been organically grown to those grown conventionally. As you can see, vegetables grown without herbicides, pesticides, and artificial fertilizers are far more nutritious.

NUTRITIONAL BENEFITS OF ORGANIC VEGETABLES
(MG EQUIVALENTS PER 100 G DRY WEIGHT)

	Calcium	Magnesium	Potassium	Sodium	Manganese	Iron	Copper
Snap Beans							
Organic	40.5	60.0	99.7	8.6	60.0	227.0	69.0
Conventional	15.5	14.8	29.1	0.0	2.0	10.0	3.0
Cabbage							
Organic	60.0	54.6	148.3	20.4	13.0	94.0	48.0
Conventional	17.5	15.6	53.7	0.8	2.0	20.0	0.4
Lettuce							
Organic	71.0	49.3	176.5	12.2	169.0	516.0	60.0
Conventional	16.0	13.1	53.7	0.0	1.0	9.0	3.0
Tomatoes							
Organic	23.0	59.2	148.3	6.5	68.0	1938.0	53.0
Conventional	4.5	4.5	58.6	0.0	1.0	1.0	0.0
Spinach							
Organic	96.0	203.9	257.0	69.5	117.0	1585.0	32.0
Conventional	47.5	46.9	84.0	0.8	1.0	19.0	0.5

Source: *Journal of Applied Nutrition*, Vol. 45, No. 1, 1983.

What Are the Benefits of Fiber?

Fiber acts as a cleanser, stimulator, and detoxifier of the gastrointestinal tract. The term "fiber" describes food residue that is not digested by the body. While the average American's intake of dietary fiber is estimated to be between 11 and 17 grams per day, it is advisable to eat more than 25 grams per day.

FIBER:

- Improves bowel function and regularity.
- Speeds up fecal transit time.
- Reduces cholesterol levels.
- May prevent and treat diverticulitis and colitis.
- May protect against colon cancer.
- May alleviate varicose veins and hemorrhoids.
- May prevent absorption of chemicals in the intestines.
- Aids in weight management.
- May assist diabetics in regulating and enhancing insulin sensitivity.
- May reduce risk of coronary heart disease.

Fiber attracts and increases the water content of fecal matter. This makes stools easier to eliminate and reduces the potential risks from toxic waste buildup in the intestinal tract. The best sources of fiber are fruit, vegetables, whole grains, beans, pasta, and cereal. Fiber is found in plant food only. There is no fiber in animal products.

What Are the Two Major Types of Fiber?

Insoluble fiber does not dissolve in water and generally passes through the intestinal tract relatively intact. Insoluble fiber components include lignin, cellulose, and hemicellulose. Soluble fiber, in contrast, dissolves in water and can be broken down by the body's intestinal bacteria. Soluble fiber, including ingredients such as pectin and guar gum, is largely responsible for the cholesterol-lowering effects of fiber. It is important to eat a variety of fiber-containing foods to obtain adequate amounts of both soluble and insoluble fiber.

TIP

- When increasing dietary fiber, increase fluid intake.
- It is important to choose a variety of high-fiber sources.
- Eat organic fruit and vegetables with the skins for highest fiber content.
- Eat five to nine servings of fruit and vegetables per day and at least 25 grams of fiber per day.
- Add ½ cup of the following into your salad to increase fiber content:

  - kidney beans (6 grams)
  - pinto beans (5 grams)
  - peas (4 grams)

  - corn (3 grams)
  - zucchini (3 grams)
  - sweet potatoes (3 grams)

Do You Know Which Is Higher in Fiber: Oranges or Black-eyed Peas?

You can obtain more fiber in your diet by consuming larger amounts of fresh fruit, vegetables, whole-grain cereals and breads, or a variety of grains and dried beans. Interestingly, these plant-based foods are also devoid of cholesterol while animal-based foods, such as chicken, beef, turkey, and lamb, are devoid of all fiber and contain varying amounts of cholesterol.

As you can see in the following table, black-eyed peas have far greater amounts of soluble and insoluble fiber than oranges. The table will inform you of the amounts of fiber in some of my favorite foods. If you're wondering "where's the beef," keep in mind that foods derived from animal sources have no fiber in them at all. Therefore, foods such as beef, chicken, lamb, pork, and fish are absent from this fiber table.

FIBER CONTENT OF SOME COMMON FOODS

	Portion		Soluble Fiber (g)	Insoluble Fiber (g)
Beans				
Black-eyed peas, cooked	½	cup	5.6	6.8
Kidney beans, cooked	½	cup	2.5	3.3
Lentils, cooked	½	cup	0.9	1.1
Lima beans, cooked	½	cup	1.2	3.2
Pinto beans, cooked	½	cup	2.0	3.3
Split peas, cooked	½	cup	1.7	3.4
White beans	½	cup	3.7	4.0
Fruit				
Apple	1	whole	0.8	1.9
Banana	1	medium	0.6	1.4
Cantaloupe	¼	small	0.5	1.1
Dried figs	1	medium	0.8	2.9
Dried prunes, cooked	⅓	cup	1.6	4.1

	Portion	Soluble Fiber (g)	Insoluble Fiber (g)
Fruit (cont.)			
Grapefruit	½ medium	0.6	1.1
Orange	1 small	0.3	0.9
Peach	1 small	0.3	1.1
Pear	½ medium	0.5	2.0
Pineapple	½ cup	0.3	0.9
Raisins	1½ Tbsp.	0.2	0.7
Strawberries	½ cup	0.3	1.1
Grain Products			
Brown rice, cooked	½ cup	0.2	2.2
Cornflakes	1 cup	0.1	0.9
Oat bran, dry	⅓ cup	2.0	2.2
Regular oats, dry	⅓ cup	1.4	1.3
Spaghetti, cooked	½ cup	0.3	0.5
Whole-wheat bread	1 slice	0.3	1.1
Whole-wheat crackers	5 crackers	0.4	1.5
Whole-wheat flour	2½ Tbsp.	0.3	1.5
Vegetables			
Bean sprouts	½ cup	0.3	1.3
Beets, cooked	½ cup	0.8	1.4
Broccoli, cooked	½ cup	0.9	1.1
Brussels sprouts, cooked	½ cup	1.6	2.3
Carrots, cooked	½ cup	1.1	1.2
Cauliflower, cooked	½ cup	0.5	1.1
Celery	½ cup	0.4	0.9
Frozen asparagus, cooked	½ cup	0.6	2.7
Frozen corn, cooked	½ cup	1.7	1.8
Frozen green peas, cooked	½ cup	1.1	3.4
Green beans, cooked	½ cup	0.5	1.6
Green pepper	½ cup	0.2	0.6
Kale	½ cup	0.6	2.0
Kidney beans	½ cup	1.4	5.2
Loose-leaf lettuce	½ cup	0.3	0.3
Mushrooms	½ cup	0.3	0.6
Onion	½ cup	0.9	1.8
Peas	½ cup	0.2	2.6
Sweet potato	½ cup	1.1	1.4

Why Are Beans and Legumes So Important?

Beans or legumes are packed with nutrients that provide protein, vitamins, and minerals. Beans are especially high in B vitamins, iron, calcium, potassium, and phosphorus. They provide approximately 6–8 grams of fiber per cup. Owing to their high protein content, beans can be used as an alternative to animal protein such as meat, chicken, and fish.

Dried beans generally take quite a while to cook, usually between forty-five minutes and two hours. The precise cooking time for beans can vary quite a bit depending on numerous factors, including the length of soaking time, the simmering temperature, and the size and age of the beans. The following table will estimate the amount of cooking time and yield for a variety of different dried beans to make your cooking experience more pleasurable and tasty.

PREPARING BEANS AND LEGUMES

Legumes (1 cup dry)	Water* (cups)	Cooking Time* (hours)	Yield* (cups)	Presoak?
Aduki beans	3	1	2	yes
Black beans	4	1–1½	2	yes
Black-eyed peas	3	1–1¼	2	no
Chickpeas (garbanzo beans)	4	2½–3	2½	yes
Fava beans	3	2	2	yes
Great Northern beans	3½	1½–2	2	yes
Kidney beans	3	1½–2	2	yes
Lentils (red or brown)	3	½–¾	2¼	no
Lima beans, baby	2	1–1¼	1¾	yes
Lima beans, large	2	1–1½	1¼	yes
Mung beans	2½	1–1¼	2	no
Navy beans	3	1–2	2	yes
Pinto beans	3	1½–2½	2	yes
Split peas	3	¾–1	2¼	yes

*Approximations.

TIPS
- Store beans in lidded jar in a cool, dry place for up to one month.
- Buy beans with uniform size and color and a plump look.
- To make beans less gassy:
  Use smaller beans and soak overnight (except aduki, lentils, split pea and red lentils).
- Cook until well done.
- Add ½ inch strip of the sea vegetable wakame to boiling water.
- Add herbs and spices such as turmeric, cumin, coriander, ginger, cardamom, clove, thyme, sage, marjoram, and bay leaves.

Grains: From Granola to Groats!

Whole grains are a nourishing staple food throughout the world. They are inexpensive, simple to prepare, and are a valuable source of fiber. Combining beans and grains provides a source of complete protein. For optimal health, try to maximize your consumption of unrefined grains and minimize your intake of refined grains.

A grain contains three layers:

- Germ: the part of the kernel that sprouts when sown; the germ is rich in protein, carbohydrates, and unsaturated fats.
- Bran: the outer layer coating the endosperm, which contains the most fiber, minerals, and B vitamins.
- Endosperm: is in the kernel and contains starch and protein.

Refined grains: lack the bran and the germ and severely lack minerals, B vitamins, and fiber.
Unrefined grains: have all three layers intact and are rich in nutritional value.

WHAT ARE THE BENEFITS OF WHOLE GRAINS?

- Excellent low-fat food.
- High in protein.
- Encompasses a wide range of B vitamins.
- High in fiber.
- Devoid of cholesterol.
- High in calcium, magnesium, iron, potassium, phosphorus, and zinc.

How long do you need to cook your grains? Each specific grain requires a different amount of cooking time and water to be added. The following guidelines will help you in preparing grains.

GUIDELINES FOR PREPARING GRAINS

Grain (1 cup dry)	Water* (cups)	Cooking Time* (minutes)	Yield* (cups)
Amaranth	2½	20	2
Barley (whole)	3	45	3½
Pot	3	50	3
Pearl	2½	40	3
Buckwheat (kasha)	2	15–20	2½
Corn meal	4	25	3
Couscous	2	15	3
Hominy Grits	4	25	3
Millet	2½–3	35–40	3½
Oats (whole grain)	3½	60	3
Steel-cut	4	40	3
Rolled	1½	10	2½
Polenta	4	25	3
Rice			
Arborio	2	25	2½
Basmati	2½	30	3
Brown	2	45	3
White	2	20	3
Wild	3	60	3½
Rye berries	3	60	2½
Quinoa	2	15	3
Teff3	15–20	3	
Wheat			
Bulgur	2	20	2½
Cracked	3	35	2½
Whole-grain wheat berries	3	60	2½

*Approximations.

What Herbs Should I Use with Chicken?

Herbs are a wonderful and nutritious way to season your food. Fresh herbs can be grown outdoors in your garden, or year-round indoors in window boxes. Fresh herbs are preferable to dried herbs for their flavor and added nutritional value.

When using dried herbs, use sparingly as the flavor is much stronger. Both dry and fresh herbs are readily available from your grocer. Herbs are also a great substitute for table salt. Since adding salt to your food may contribute to high blood pressure, headaches, or water retention, consider trying some of the herbs listed below.

The following table gives you practical suggestions to enhance your meals.

Herb	Flavor	Try with
Basil	Fragrant, sweet, and mildly peppery	Tomato sauces, salad dressing, poultry, fish, soups, and casseroles
Chervil	Mild, parsley-like flavor	Egg and fish dishes, sauces, and salads
Chives	Mild, sweet onion taste	Egg, cheese, vegetable dishes, soups, and salads
Cilantro (fresh coriander)	Distinctive pungent grassy flavor	Poultry, fish, vegetables and sauces; with avocado, corn, or black beans
Coriander (seed)	Strong sage flavor with a citrus bite	Chicken, beets, onion, chilies, curries, and chutneys
Dill	Slightly sweet with sharp tang	Fish, eggs, carrots, cauliflower, spinach, cheeses, potatoes, yogurt dips, or sauce
Fennel	Soft, nutty, anise/celery flavor	Fish, cabbage, soup, salads, breads
Marjoram	Mild oregano taste	Stuffing, lamb, beef, vegetable dishes, casseroles, and soups
Mint	Cool, refreshing, sweet	Tea, yogurt, fruit, carrots, peas
Oregano	Pungent, peppery, slightly bitter	Pizza, tomatoes, mushrooms, poultry, lentils
Parsley	Mild leafy flavor	Chicken, beef, shellfish, pasta, sauces, egg dishes, and casseroles
Rosemary	Pine-like fragrance, savory yet sweet	Roasted vegetables, grain dishes, fish, meat, poultry, soups
Sage	Pleasantly tart, lemony zest	Breads, stuffing, potatoes, pork, and duck
Savory	Light, sweet with a pepper tang	Beans, lentils, vegetables, meat loaf, and tea
Sorrel	Lemon-like or sour taste	Spinach, cabbage, lettuce, fish, salads, sauces, and coleslaw
Tarragon	Anise-like	Chicken, fish, veal, young vegetables, and sauces
Thyme	Pleasant, fresh taste with faint clove aftertaste	Veal, lamb, poultry, salad dressing, stuffings, and casseroles

Sea Vegetables: See the Benefits from the Sea!

Sea vegetables have the highest nutritive potency of any source of food. Sea vegetables are an important component of a macrobiotic diet and can be purchased in health food stores and some supermarkets. Gradually introducing small amounts of sea vegetables to your diet can greatly improve your health status.

WHAT ARE THE BENEFITS OF SEA VEGETABLES?

Sea vegetables:

- Improve skin tone.
- Prevent wrinkles.
- Improve hair quality.
- Purify the blood.
- Dissolve fat and mucus.
- Neutralize radioactive materials.
- Alkalinize the body.
- Supply fiber to digestive system.

Sea vegetables, which have been associated with the Japanese diet, are also being incorporated more into the American diet of late. Some may also use the term "seaweed" or "marine algae" when referring to these nourishing foods. They contain high sources of vitamins and minerals, including significant amounts of calcium, iron, phosphorus, magnesium, iodine, zinc, copper, and fluoride. The B vitamins—thiamine, niacin, riboflavin, folic acid, B_6 and B_{12}—along with vitamins A, C, E, and K, can all be found in different sea vegetables. These foods are also very low in fat and their calorie content is almost negligible. Most sea vegetables come from coastal regions of waterways including oceans, bays, inlets, and peninsulas.

Sea vegetables are generally purchased in a dried form and most commonly sold in health food stores in sealed cellophane packages. They are quite resistant to spoilage and can last up to two years if stored in a tightly sealed jar, preferably in a cool, dry place.

The following will describe a few of the more commonly used and versatile sea vegetables that you may wish to add to your diet.

What Is Agar?

Agar has a gelling-like effect. It can be purchased either in bars tightly wrapped in cellophane or in flakes. It has virtually no calories and is high in fiber. It can be used to yield a colorless, odorless, and flavorless gelatin. One tablespoon of agar flakes will gel one cup of liquid while one agar bar will gel up to three cups of liquid. If using the bar, break it into several pieces and combine it with liquid in a saucepan. Bring to a boil and then simmer for fifteen minutes, stirring occasionally. If using the flakes, bring the liquid to a boil, sprinkle in the flakes, and then simmer for two to three minutes, stirring occasionally.

You can use this with fruit juice, vegetable juice, or bouillon, along with other flavorings or solid ingredients. Then allow the dish to chill thoroughly and refrigerate for at least two hours. Once chilled, the consistency will resemble that of pudding.

TIP

Do not use agar in the presence of vinegar, chocolate, or spinach. Certain substances contained within these foods will interfere with the gelling action of agar. If mixed with pineapple or tomato juice, agar may not set as firmly as with other liquids.

What Is Arame?

Arame is cooked after being harvested and then sun-dried. When purchased, it will appear almost black in color in short strands. It needs to be reconstituted prior to use. Simply soak it for approximately five minutes in warm water before adding it to your recipe. It can be added to your favorite spaghetti sauce and served over hot pasta. You can also consider adding it to hot and sour soup or vegetable and noodle soups.

What Is Dulse?

Dulse has a tangy, salty flavor and is 22 percent protein. It is quite versatile and can be used either straight from the package, toasted, or reconstituted. Some prefer to use it simply from the package as a snack, either plain or dipped in yogurt. It can be used as a substitute for bacon in a lettuce and tomato sandwich. In order to do this, dulse should be toasted in a moderately hot, dry skillet until it becomes a dull brownish-green. You could also crumble the toasted dulse and sprinkle it as a seasoning over a green salad or noodle dishes. Hot and cold dulse can also be reconstituted by soaking it in lukewarm water for five minutes. You can then add it to a recipe calling for cooked spinach, chard, or collard greens and substitute about one-quarter of the amount called for with reconstituted dulse. Be aware that its volume will increase two to three times when reconstituted.

What is Hijiki?

Hijiki has a strong ocean flavor and is probably the most difficult sea vegetable to acquire a taste for. It is usually sold in packages as small dark, curly pieces. Its calcium content is extraordinary. Just one tablespoon of hijiki provides fourteen times more calcium than a cup of milk. Hijiki will also expand to four times its volume when reconstituted. Simply soak it in warm water for ten to fifteen minutes. You can try using a small amount of reconstituted hijiki to garnish a hot grain or noodle dish.

A traditional Japanese recipe for hijiki includes heating two tablespoons of peanut oil in a skillet and then adding one large chopped onion, one large, thinly sliced carrot, one cup of grated daikon radish, and one cup of reconstituted hijiki. Sauté until all the vegetables are golden and then season with soy sauce and lemon juice or rice vinegar.

What are Kombu and Kelp?

Kombu and kelp have similar flavors and usages. They are usually a dark olive green and packaged in wide flat pieces. You can reconstitute kombu and kelp by cutting four- to five-inch lengths and soaking in warm water for five to ten minutes. They can then be cut into strips or small squares and added to stir-fry vegetables, stews, soups, or hot grain dishes. You may find it tasty to add noodles flavored with miso or soy sauce.

What is Nori?

Nori can be purchased in dark purplish or olive brown sheets wrapped in cellophane packages in a natural food store or Asian grocery store. You may be familiar with sushi that is wrapped with nori. It is extremely high in protein content, at 35 percent, and it is as abundant in vitamin A as carrots. It also contains enzymes to assist digestion. Unlike other sea vegetables, nori is not reconstituted but toasted. You can use nori to wrap rice or sushi. Alternatively, you can cut the toasted nori sheets into two-inch strips and wrap pieces of tofu or cucumber along with rice.

What is Wakame?

Wakame is a dark green, long-leafed sea vegetable that has a mild flavor and can be used similarly to kombu. It comes in long strands, approximately two inches wide. To reconstitute, simply tear off the desired amount and soak in warm water for ten minutes. It will also expand to two or three times its volume. Try adding a small amount of chopped reconstituted wakame and scallions to scrambled eggs. This will help to increase your intake of calcium, phosphorus, and iron. You can also try adding it to split pea soup or to miso soup.

What nutrients are found in the sea vegetables? As you can see from the following table, sea vegetables are generally high in protein, calcium, iron, phosphorus, and B vitamins.

Sea Vegetable	High In
Agar	Fiber, vitamins A, B_1, B_6, B_{12}, C, D, K, and biotin. Aids intestinal action, binds with radioactive and toxic wastes to carry them out of the body.
Arame	Protein, potassium, iron, calcium, iodine, phosphorus, vitamins A, B_1, and B_2.
Dulse	Iron, protein, calcium, phosphorus, iodine, potassium, magnesium, vitamins A, C, B_6, B_{12}, and E.
Hijiki	Calcium, phosphorus, iron, protein, and vitamins A and B_2.
Kombu	Protein, iron, calcium, phosphorus, vitamins A, B_2, and C. Good for high blood pressure, weight control, and anemia; cleanses colon; aids kidneys.
Nori	Protein, calcium, iron, potassium, magnesium, phosphorus, iodine; very high in vitamins A, B_2, C, D, and niacin. Lowers cholesterol, aids digestion.
Wakame	Protein, iron, calcium, magnesium, phosphorus; large amounts of vitamin C, plus B_{12}, A, B_2, and niacin.

Can Proper Food Combining Reduce Intestinal Gas and Bloating?

Some individuals notice that they feel better when they combine foods in a particular fashion. They may also notice that certain combinations of foods contribute to intestinal gas, bloating, or cramping. Proper food combining may help to reduce intestinal gas and bloating and assist with good digestion and assimilation. Although a food-combining diet is not for everyone, it may be worth experimenting with should you have gastrointestinal complaints.

Some of my patients have reported that they had more intestinal symptoms when they combined proteins and starches, yet they could eat them separately without obvious problems. Others have found that difficulty with weight loss could be solved by following food-combining principles. You might want to experiment with this diet for a few weeks to see whether or not your digestion becomes more efficient.

The following recommendations may be helpful in following a food-combining diet:

Food Combining Do's and Don'ts

Do:

- Combine any protein, including fish, chicken, or meat, along with any leafy or starchy vegetables. For example, you may combine a piece of flounder or chicken along with spinach or carrots.
- Combine starches (such as beans, grains, corn, potatoes or squash) with leafy or starchy vegetables (such as carrots, peas, cauliflower, onions or garlic). For example, combining rice and beans along with onions and asparagus would be acceptable.
- Eat melons alone and not combined with any other foods.
- Eat acid and subacid fruits (such as apples, apricots, peaches, cherries and oranges) alone. They can also be combined with nuts and seeds.
- Eat sweet fruits (such as bananas, dates, figs, raisins and grapes) after acid or subacid fruits, or alone.
- Consume dairy products alone or combined with grains or green nonstarchy vegetables (such as broccoli, spinach, green beans and peppers).
- Eat fruits at least two hours before or after all other foods.

Don't:

- Combine proteins and starches at the same meal.
- Mix fruits with other foods, especially proteins.
- Combine vegetables and fruit at the same meal.

Tips For Healthier Eating

These recommendations will help you achieve a better diet. Use them as dietary goals which you will reach in time by changing your current diet.

Do:

- Take time and effort to obtain healthy food.
- Take time and effort to prepare a variety of foods that are palatable and nutritious.
- Take time to eat slowly and enjoy the food you are eating.
- Eat numerous smaller meals and healthy snacks.

Avoid:

- Processed food
- Sugar
- Alcohol
- Caffeine
- White flour products
- Hydrogenated fats
- Chemicals
- Aluminum and Teflon cookware
- Salt
- Nonorganic meat and produce
- Spoiled fruit, vegetables, and grains

Food Preparation:

- Eat fruits and vegetables as soon as possible after picking.
- Cut vegetables into large pieces for cooking; small pieces have greater surface area exposed, resulting in greater nutrient loss.
- Use a vegetable steamer; boiling destroys nutrients.
- Undercook rather than overcook to avoid nutrient loss.
- Use lower heat to prepare vegetables; the higher the heat, the greater the nutrient loss.
- Eat raw fruit and vegetables to gain optimum nutrient value.
- Rinse grains quickly before cooking to remove dirt and sediment; avoid overrinsing.
- Use cooking water as an excellent source of nutrients for soups, sauces, or juices.

CHAPTER 7

Foods and Substances to Avoid

Potentially harmful substances—or foods that have been processed to the point of removing vital nutrients—should be avoided as often as possible. Although this may be difficult (particularly since some of these substances, such as caffeine, wine, and cigarettes can be addictive), the benefits that will result will bring new vitality and health to the reader.

Why Should I Avoid Refined or Processed Foods?

Processing or refining foods involves the removal of the key nutritious elements of a food in an effort to make the food easier to cook, faster to prepare or longer lasting on the shelf. In doing so, most of the food's original vitamins and minerals, as well as fiber content, are stripped away. To compensate for the removal of key nutrients, a host of additives, preservatives, and enhancers are added back to the product. Most of these "extras" are from additional fats or chemicals that may be potentially hazardous to your health. These so-called "extras" generally will increase the fat content of your food and are generally devoid of health-enhancing vitamins, minerals, and fiber. On the other hand, you may have adverse reactions to the artificial chemicals, food colorings, dyes, or preservatives that are frequently added to processed foods. Some of these "extras" are added to foods to extend shelf life, appearance, or possibly flavor.

I am also quite concerned about the long-term health effects that these nonnutritious foods might have over the years. It is my belief that eating too many processed foods can increase your susceptibility to developing heart disease, hypertension, obesity, colitis, fatigue, and even cancer.

VITAMIN AND MINERAL LOSSES IN THE REFINING OF WHOLE WHEAT INTO FLOUR

Vitamin	% Lost	Mineral	% Lost
B$_1$ (thiamine)	77	Chromium	40
B$_2$ (riboflavin)	80	Manganese	90
B$_3$ (niacin)	81	Copper	68
B$_6$ (pyridoxine)	72	Zinc	78
Pantothenic acid	50	Iron	81
Folic acid	67	Magnesium	85
Vitamin E	86		

Our best sources of high-quality carbohydrates, proteins, fats, vitamins, and minerals are whole, unprocessed, unpackaged, or minimally packaged foods. Fresh fruit and vegetables, grains, beans, or legumes should be the basis of our diet. The following table lists the substantial nutrient losses which occur when refining whole wheat into white flour. As you can see from the table on page 82, nearly 70–80 percent of most of the important vitamins and minerals that your body requires are removed during this refining process.

What Is a Food Additive?

Food additives are substances or a combination of substances that are widely used in the processing and storage of many foods. There are over 10,000 food additives in use in our food supply today. Food additives are used to preserve food, inhibit mold and fungal growth, retard food spoilage, and prevent color changes.

Adverse reactions to food additives may be immediate or delayed. If you have adverse reactions to food additives, you may need to avoid them completely. Read food labels to select additive-free foods.

SYMPTOMS OF ADVERSE REACTIONS TO FOOD ADDITIVES:

- Asthma
- Faintness
- Hives
- Irritable bowel
- Runny nose

- Bleeding
- Headaches
- Hyperactivity
- Nasal polyps
- Skin eruptions

- Dermatitis
- Heart palpitations
- Irritability
- Rhinitis
- Swelling

COMMON FOOD ADDITIVES

Food Additive	Description
Alginate	Thickening agent and foam stabilizer. Used in ice cream, cheese, candy, and yogurt.
Propylene glycol	Made from seaweed.
Artificial flavoring	Used in soda pop, candy, breakfast cereals, gelatin, and many other foods.
Ascorbic acid	Antioxidant, nutrient, color stabilizer.
Aspartame	Artificial sweetener in drink mixes, gelatin, candy, diet beverages, and other foods.
Blue No. 1	Coloring in beverages, candy and baked goods. Small cancer risk.
Blue No. 2	Coloring in pet food, beverages, and candy. Small cancer risk in mice.
Brominated vegetable oil (BVO)	Emulsifier, clouding agent in soft drinks.
Butylated hydroxytoluene (BHT)	Antioxidant in cereals, chewing gum, potato chips, oils, and other foods.
Calcium propionate	Preservative in bakery goods.
Calcium stearyl lactylate	Dough conditioner. Whipping agent in bread dough, cake fillings, artificial whipping cream, and processed egg whites.
Carrageenan	Thickening and stabilizing agent in ice cream, jelly, chocolate milk, and infant formula.
Casein, sodium caseinate	Thickening and whitening agent in ice cream, coffee creamers, and sherbet.
Citric acid, sodium citrate	Acid flavoring, chelating agent in ice cream, sherbet, fruit drink, candy, soda, and instant potatoes.
Citrus red No. 2 orange	Coloring in skin of some Florida oranges. Dye does not leach through skin.
Corn syrup	Sweetener, thickener in candy toppings, syrups, snack foods, and imitation dairy products.
Dextrose (glucose, corn sugar)	Sweetener, coloring agent in bread, caramel, soda, cookies, and other foods.
EDTA	Chelating agent in salad dressings, margarine, sandwich spreads, mayonnaise, processed fruits and vegetables, canned shellfish, and soda.
Erythorbic acid	Antioxidant and color stabilizer in oily foods, cereals, soft drinks, and cured meats.
Ferrous gluconate	Coloring, nutrient in black olives.
Fumaric acid	Tartness agent in powdered drinks, pudding, pie filling, and gelatin.
Gelatin	Thickening and gelling agent in powdered drinks, pudding, pie filling, and gelatin.

Food Additive	Description
Glycerin (glycerol)	Maintains water content in marshmallows, candy, fudge, and baked goods.
Green No. 3	Coloring in candy, beverages. Small cancer risk.
Gums	Thickening agent and stabilizer in beverages, ice cream, frozen pudding, salad dressing, dough, cottage cheese, candy, and drink mixes.
Heptyl paraben	Preservative in beer and noncarbonated soft drinks.
Hydrogenated vegetable oil	Source of oil in margarine, many processed foods.
Hydrolyzed vegetable protein (HVP)	Flavor enhancer in instant soups, frankfurters, sauce mixes, and beef stew.
Invert sugar	Sweetener in candy, sodas, and many other foods.
Lactic acid	Acidity regulator in Spanish olives, cheese, frozen desserts, and carbonated beverages.
Lactose	Sweetener in whipped-topping mix and breakfast pastries.
Lecithin	Emulsifier, antioxidant in baked goods, margarine, chocolate, and ice cream.
Mannitol	Sweetener in chewing gum and low-calorie foods.
Monoglycerides, Diglycerides	Emulsifier in baked goods, margarine, candy, and peanut butter.
Monosodium gluconate (MSG)	Flavor enhancer in soup, seafood, poultry, cheese, sauces, stews, and other foods.
Phosphoric acid	Acidifier, chelating agent in butter, emulsifier, nutrient-discoloration inhibitor in cheese, powdered foods, cured meat, soda, baked goods, breakfast cereals, and dehydrated potatoes.
Polysorbate 60	Emulsifier in baked goods, frozen desserts, and imitation dairy products.
Propyl gallate	Antioxidant in vegetable oil, meat products, potato sticks, chicken soup base, and chewing gum.
Quinine	Flavoring in tonic water, quinine water, and bitter lemon.
Red No. 3	Coloring in cherries, candy, and baked goods. Cancer risk.
Red No. 40	Coloring in soda, candy, gelatin desserts, pastry, pet food, and sausage.
Saccharin	Synthetic sweetener in diet products.
Sodium benzoate	Preservative in fruit juice, carbonated drinks, pickles, and preserves.
Sodium carboxyl methylcellulose	Thickening and stabilizing agent in ice cream, beer, pie fillings, icings, diet foods, and candy.

Food Additive	Description
Sodium nitrite, nitrate	Preservative, coloring, flavoring used in bacon, ham, frankfurters, luncheon meats, smoked fish, and corned beef.
Sorbic acid, potassium sorbate	Prevents growth of mold in cheese, syrup, jelly, cake, wine, and dry fruits.
Sorbitan monostearate	Emulsifier in cakes, candy, frozen pudding, and icings.
Sorbitol	Sweetener, thickening agent in dietetic drinks and food, candy, shredded coconut, and chewing gum.
Starch, modified	Thickening agent in soup, gravy, and baby foods.
Sulfur dioxide, sodium bisulfite sulfite	Preservative and bleach used in sliced fruit, wine, and processed potatoes. May cause severe allergic reactions in certain people, especially asthmatics.
Vanillin, ethyl vanillin	Substitute for vanilla in ice cream, baked goods, beverages, chocolate, candy, and gelatin.
Yellow No. 5 (Tartrazine)	Coloring in gelatin, candy, pet food, baked goods. May cause allergic reactions.
Yellow No. 6	Coloring in beverages, sausage, baked goods, candy. Cancer risk.

Beware of Sulfites

Sulfites are often added to foods to function as an antioxidant to help preserve the foods from spoiling. Sulfites may be labeled as sulfur dioxide, metabisulfite, or sodium bisulfite. Many people, particularly those with asthma, can have allergic reactions to sulfites. Others have also reported headaches, dizziness, blurred vision, or shortness of breath. All efforts should be made to avoid sulfites.

COMMON FOODS WITH SULFITES

Food Category	Types of Food
Alcoholic beverages	Wine, beer, cocktail mixes, wine coolers, most distilled liquors.
Baked goods	Bread with dough conditioners, cookies, crackers, crepes, mixes, pie crust, pizza crust, quiche crust, soft pretzels, tortillas and tortilla shells, waffles.
Beverage bases and nonalcoholic beverages	Most beverages containing sugar and/or corn syrup; dried citrus fruit beverage mixes; all canned, bottled, or frozen fruit juices.
Condiments and relishes	Horseradish, onion and pickle relishes, pickles, olives, salad dressing mixes, wine vinegar.
Confections and frostings	Most canned or packaged frosting mixes.
Dairy product analogs	Most processed "cheese foods" containing "filled milk," skim milk enriched in fat content by addition of vegetable oils.
Dried seasonigs	Chives, parsley, herbs, and spices.
Fish and shellfish (fresh)	Shrimp, scallops.
Shellfish (processed–frozen, canned, and dried)	Clams, shrimp, lobster, crab, scallops, dried cod.
Gelatins, puddings, fillings	Fruit fillings, flavored and unflavored gelatin, pectin, jelling agents.
Grain products and pasta	Cornstarch, modified food starch, spinach pasta, gravies, breadings, batters, noodle and rice mixes.
Hard candies	Most clear, hard candy.
Jams and jellies	Most jams and jellies.
Nuts and nut products	Shredded coconut.
Processed fruits	Most dried fruit, including raisins and prunes; canned, bottled, or frozen fruit; maraschino cherries; glazed fruit.
Processed vegetables	Vegetable juices; canned vegetables (including potatoes); pickled vegetables (including sauerkraut, cauliflower, and peppers); dried vegetables; instant mashed potatoes; all frozen vegetables, including french fries; deli potato salad.
Refined sugar	Most sugar–brown, white, powdered, and raw.
Snack foods	Dried fruit snacks, trail mixes, filled crackers, tortilla chips, potato chips.
Soups and soup mixes	Canned soups, dried soup mixes.
Sweet sauces, toppings, syrups	Corn syrup, maple syrup, fruit toppings, high-fructose corn syrup, pancake syrup, molasses.
Tea	Instant tea, liquid tea concentrates.

Don't Overdose on Caffeine

Caffeine is the world's most prevalent drug, and it is commonly found in coffee, tea, colas, chocolate, and some medications. Caffeine is addictive and stimulates the central nervous system, cardiac muscle, and gastric secretions. As little as one cup of coffee can trigger erratic blood sugar reactions in some individuals, stimulating the adrenal glands, and thereby causing the liver to release more sugar into the bloodstream. Consumed in large quantities, caffeine can reduce the level of calcium in bones, leading to osteoporosis. Many people consuming large quantities of caffeine (through coffee, colas, and chocolates) suffer a caffeine-induced blood pressure elevation and rapid heart rate. Interestingly, women who consume caffeine can experience a worsening of benign breast cysts and premenstrual syndrome.

Recently, drinking more than three cups of coffee per day has been shown to lessen a woman's chance of becoming pregnant. And drinking as little as two or three cups per day can increase a pregnant woman's risk of delivering an underweight baby, one with a birth defect, or possibly even cause a miscarriage. As a result, women who are trying to become pregnant or who are currently pregnant should consume as little caffeine as possible. When attempting to eliminate caffeine from your diet, you may experience a variety of withdrawal symptoms such as headaches, fatigue, and depression.

What Are the Symptoms of Excessive Caffeine?

- Chronic anxiety
- Gastric acid secretion
- Heart palpitations
- Insomnia
- Light-headedness
- Muscle twitches

The amount of caffeine in any given drink depends on several factors; for example, the type of coffee or tea you drink, how it's brewed, and of course, the size of your coffee mug. Furthermore, the amount of caffeine contained in regular brewed coffee, espresso, and other designer coffees can vary greatly. The following table indicates the approximate amount of caffeine in a variety of different beverages and medications.

COMMON SOURCES OF CAFFEINE

Product	Serving Size	Caffeine (mg)
OTC Drugs		
NoDoz, maximum strength; Vivarin	1 tablet	200
Excedrin	2 tablets	130
NoDoz, regular strength	1 tablet	100
Anacin	2 tablets	64

Product	Serving Size	Caffeine (mg)
Coffees		
Coffee, brewed	8 oz	135
General Foods International Coffee, Orange Cappuccino	8 oz	102
Coffee, instant	8 oz	95
General Foods International Coffee, Cafe Vienna	8 oz	90
Maxwell House Cappuccino, Mocha	8 oz	60–65
General Foods International Coffee, Swiss Mocha	8 oz	55
Maxwell House Cappuccino, French Vanilla or Irish Cream	8 oz	45–50
Maxwell House Cappuccino, Amaretto	8 oz	25–30
General Foods International Coffee, Viennese Chocolate Cafe	8 oz	26
Maxwell House Cappuccino, decaffeinated	8 oz	3–6
Teas		
Celestial Seasonings Iced Lemon Ginseng Tea	16 oz bottle	100
Bigelow Raspberry Royale Tea	8 oz	83
Tea, leaf or bag	8 oz	50
Snapple Iced Tea, all varieties	16 oz bottle	48
Lipton Natural Brew Iced Tea Mix, Unsweetened	8 oz	25–45
Lipton Tea	8 oz	35–40
Lipton Natural Brew Iced Tea Mix, Sweetened	8 oz	15–35
Tea, green	8 oz	30
Arizona Iced Tea, assorted varieties	16 oz bottle	15–30
Tea, instant	8 oz	15
Lipton Natural Brew Iced Tea Mix, diet	8 oz	10–15
Lipton Natural Brew Iced Tea Mix, decaffeinated	8 oz	<5
Celestial Seasonings Herbal Tea, all varieties	8 oz	0
Celestial Seasonings Herbal Iced Tea, bottled	16 oz bottle	0
Lipton Soothing Moments Peppermint Tea	8 oz	0
Soft Drinks		
Mountain Dew	12 oz	58
Diet Coke	12 oz	51
Coca-Cola	12 oz	45
Dr. Pepper, regular or diet	12 oz	41
Sunkist Orange Soda	12 oz	40
Pepsi-Cola	12 oz	37
Barqs Root Beer	12 oz	23
7-Up or Diet 7-Up	12 oz	0
Caffeine-free Coca-Cola or Diet Coke	12 oz	0
Caffeine-free Pepsi or Diet Pepsi	12 oz	0
Sprite or Diet Sprite	12 oz	0

Sources: National Coffee Associates, National Soft Drink Association, Tea Council of the USA, and *Food Chemistry and Toxicology*, 43:119, 1996.

Must I Stop Smoking?

Yes. It is now well documented that smoking is hazardous to your health. Adverse health effects include cancer, heart disease, hypertension, oxygen deprivation, respiratory infections, emphysema, and low infant birthweight. There is further evidence that cigarette smoking can cause free radicals to form in your body, thereby damaging even more of your cells. Even being exposed to secondhand smoke can be detrimental to your health. If you cannot quit completely, try to reduce the number of cigarettes you smoke each day and set a target date for when you hope to stop completely. Be aware that you may experience withdrawal symptoms when you reduce your smoking.

Cigarette Withdrawal Symptoms Include:

- Headaches
- Body aches
- Depression
- Anxiety

Treatment for Smoking Cessation May Include:

- Herbal remedies containing lobelia, skullcap, and passion flower.
- Nutritional supplements including vitamin C, vitamin B complex, pantothenic acid (B_5), niacinamide, calcium, and magnesium.
- Acupuncture, hypnosis, biofeedback, behavior modification, and guided imagery to help reduce cravings.
- A healthy dose of desire and willpower.
- Patches that are now available both over-the-counter and by prescription.

Why Is Excessive Alcohol Consumption Dangerous?

In 1966, alcoholism was officially recognized by the American Medical Association as a disease. It is estimated that 8–12 percent of the adult population is dependent on alcohol. Although excessive alcohol consumption may be hazardous, studies have shown that small quantities of red wine may be beneficial owing to its flavonoids, a potent class of antioxidants.

Effects of excessive alcohol consumption and alcohol-induced diseases include liver disease, mental confusion, irritability, anorexia, malnutrition, hypoglycemia, vitamin and mineral deficiencies, and leaky gut syndrome. Alcohol decreases absorption and utilization of nutrients, in particular, vitamin B_{12}, folic acid, thiamine (B_1), and magnesium. It may also create electrolyte imbalances and promote night blindness. Alcohol also creates risks for people having surgery. These risks include delayed wound healing, and liver failure.

Alcohol is known to thin blood. It is implicated in reducing clotting and promoting nosebleeds. One study found that men who drink as little as three to four beers per day had a higher incidence of chronic nosebleeds than men who consumed fewer than five beers per week.

Because many chemical additives are used in various alcoholic drinks, alcohol increases the potential for food allergies and food intolerances. Therefore, it is advisable to limit alcohol intake, to be aware of possible "hidden" food allergies (as described on page 148), and to devise a program to supplement possible nutrient deficiencies induced by alcohol consumption.

CHAPTER 8

Special Diets

One man's meat is another man's poison.
—Lucretius

Diet plays a major role in achieving and maintaining optimal health. Do we all need to be on the same exact diet? Probably not. Since each individual has different biochemical and metabolic needs, it is important to select the diet that is best for you. As your biochemical and metabolic needs, desires, and goals change, your dietary choices may need to be altered. You may wish to consult with your health-care practitioner as to which specific diet may be the most beneficial to you.

The Cardiovascular Disease Reversal Diet

Cardiovascular disease is the number one cause of death in developed nations. The Cardiovascular Disease Reversal Diet was designed to help reverse cardiovascular disease. There have been hundreds of reported success stories using this diet.

Although there may be differing opinions as to the most effective diet to reverse cardiovascular disease, the consensus of most medical authorities is that a low-fat, high-fiber, vegetarian-based diet may be the most effective. This diet has also been found to improve athletic performance, promote weight loss, reduce the risk of cancer, reduce cholesterol levels, and lower blood pressure.

Several doctors have suggested that all sources of animal protein, such as milk, butter, eggs, cheese, meat, chicken, turkey, pork, and veal be limited and ideally excluded to get rid of plaque buildup. They emphasize the judicious intake of foods such as whole grains, beans, legumes, pasta, fruit, and vegetables.

It is possible to reverse heart disease. To do so, start with a diet that is particularly low in saturated fats (especially those derived from animal sources), low in cholesterol, and low in processed food, sugar, and salt. In contrast, the cardiovascular disease reversal diet should be particularly plentiful in fresh vegetables, a variety of legumes combined with whole grains, fresh fruit, and soy-based protein. You should greatly curtail your intake of all sources of animal protein, including milk, butter, eggs, cheese, meat, chicken, turkey, pork, and veal.

Following this type of diet can help to reduce the amount of atherosclerosis or plaque that may have built up in your arteries. When excess amounts of plaque accumulate in your blood vessels, blood flow becomes restricted and compromised. You are then prone to symptoms such as chest pains, shortness of breath, stroke, or even a heart attack.

To make the cardiovascular disease reversal diet most effective, I also suggest combining it with exercise, a regular stress reduction program, and specific nutritional supplements and antioxidants.

FOODS PERMITTED FOR CARDIOVASCULAR DISEASE REVERSAL DIET

Fruits	Animal Products	Whole Grains	Beverages	Legumes	Vegetables	
Apples	Egg whites	Amaranth	Club soda	Adzuki beans	Artichokes	Sprouts
Apricots	Nonfat milk	Barley	Fruit juices	Black beans	Asparagus	Squash
Bananas	Yogurt	Buckwheat	Grain coffees	Black-eyed peas	Bamboo	Sweet potatoes
Blackberries		Bulgur	Herbal teas	Brown beans	shoots	Swiss chard
Blueberries		Corn	Mineral water	Chickpeas	Beets	Turnips
Cantaloupes		Millet	Vegetable juices	(garbanzos)	Broccoli	Watercress
Casaba melons		Oats		Great Northern	Brussels	Yams
Cherries		Quinoa		beans	sprouts	Zucchini
Cranberries		Rice		Kidney beans	Cabbage	
Currants		Rye		Lentils	Carrots	
Dates		Sorghum		Mung beans	Cauliflower	
Figs		Teff		Navy beans	Celery	
Grapefruit		Wheat		Peas	Chili peppers	
Grapes				Pinto beans	Collards	
Guava				Red Mexican	Cucumbers	
Honeydew melons				beans	Eggplant	
Kiwis				Soybeans	Escarole	
Kumquats				(including	Garlic	
Lemons				tofu, miso,	Gingerroot	
Limes				and tempeh)	Jerusalem	
Loganberries					artichoke	
Mangoes					Jicama	
Nectarines					Kale	
Oranges					Leeks	
Papaya					Lettuce	
Peaches					Mushrooms	
Pears					Mustard greens	
Pineapples					Okra	
Plantains					Onions	
Plums					Parsley	
Pomegranates					Potatoes	
Prunes					Pumpkin	
Raisins					Radishes	
Raspberries					Rutabagas	
Strawberries					Scallions	
Tangelos					Shallots	
Tangerines					Sorrel	
Tomatoes					Spinach	
Watermelon						

Food Allergies and Diet

There are various diets to detect whether your symptoms are due to food allergy. Unfortunately, the diagnosis of food allergy is not easy. Because we eat a variety of foods at any one meal, it may be difficult to detect which food is actually causing the allergic response. The symptoms of food allergy may appear similar to those caused by other medical conditions.

There are several different diets that are helpful in either diagnosing and/or treating food sensitivities. Some have found that rotating these problem foods or eating them less frequently is all that may be necessary to eliminate adverse reactions. Others have found that completely avoiding the problem-causing food is imperative. Some of the most common allergies include dairy, wheat, corn, soy, eggs, yeast, and gluten products.

Symptoms of Food Allergies

Food allergies or simply being sensitive to foods are perhaps one of the most common causes of undiagnosed symptoms. You may experience chronic fatigue, frequent headaches, intestinal gas or bloating, ongoing depression, or joint pain and swelling triggered by specific foods in your diet. Not all food allergies come on immediately to cause, for example, hives, itching, or a swollen throat. More commonly, food allergies may be noted two to four hours (or even more) after eating the offending food.

For example, extreme fatigue and mental fogginess may develop soon after eating your morning bowl of cereal. Your problem may not be insufficient sleep, but sensitivity to the milk or wheat you recently ingested. Or if you notice that after ingesting beef or hamburgers on a frequent basis, your joints swell or are painful, you might be suffering from allergic arthritis.

Obviously in these cases, modify your diet either to limit the intake of the offending food or to completely avoid it for a period of time. You might find that you feel best if you design a diet that varies your food selections and allows you to eat them on a rotational basis, perhaps once every four days instead of every day as per your current diet.

Rotation Diet

A rotation diet may be used for both diagnosis and treatment of food allergies or sensitivities. This diet may be difficult to comply with but can be an important aspect of treatment for food sensitivities. It has been estimated that Americans get 80 percent of their calories from only twenty different foods, depriving themselves of a well-rounded nutritional content. It is advisable to incorporate a variety of foods into your diet, rotating them for maximal health benefit. Many have found that following a rotation diet also assists in weight loss.

Instituting a Rotation Diet

On a rotation diet, foods that you are allergic to are either eaten on a limited basis or are completely avoided for a period of time. All other foods are then ingested on a less frequent basis, commonly every fourth day. For example, if you eat chicken on Monday, you should not repeat eating it again until Friday, four days later. Likewise, if you have an apple for a snack on Tuesday, you should not snack on apples again until Saturday night, also four days later.

However, foods that are closely related (i.e., members of the same biological food family) should be ingested only every other day. For example, since pears and apples are both in the "pomme" family, you should probably wait until Thursday (in the above scenario) before eating pears.

While food allergies certainly don't cause all medical problems, they are an all-too-common trigger of many chronic undiagnosed clinical symptoms. For this reason, I make food sensitivities a top priority when I consult with patients who have a variety of ongoing, undiagnosed complaints. Food allergies can affect virtually every organ system of the body.

Making selections based on the various food families is essential in following a rotation diet. Use the following table as a guideline when making selections from the various food groups.

FOOD FAMILIES FOR A ROTATION DIET

Grass (Grains)
Barley: malt, maltose
Bamboo shoots
Corn: (mature) corn meal, corn oil, cornstarch, corn sugar, corn syrup, hominy grits, popcorn
Lemon grass, citronella
Millet
Oat, oatmeal
Rice, rice flour
Rye
Sorghum grain syrup, cane sugar, molasses, raw sugar
Sweet corn
Triticale
Wheat: bran, bulgur, flour gluten, graham, patent, whole wheat, wheat germ
Wild rice

Mustard
Broccoli
Brussels sprouts
Cabbage
Cauliflower
Celery
Collard
Horseradish
Kale
Kohlrabi
Mustard
Turnip
Rutabaga
Radish
Watercress

Plants
Carrot
Celery
Caraway
Anise
Dill
Fennel
Coriander
Cumin
Chervil
Parsley
Parsnip

Sunflower
Jerusalem artichoke
Sunflower seed oil

Walnut
Butternut
Hickory nut
Pecan
Walnut, black
Walnut, English

Pepper
Black pepper

Nutmeg
Nutmeg

Cashew
Cashew
Mango
Pistachio

Grapes
Grape brandy, champagne, cream of tartar, dried currants, raisins, wine, wine vinegar muscadine

Mollusks
Abalone
Clam
Mussel
Oyster
Scallop
Squid

Fish
All types

Crustaceans
Crab
Crayfish
Lobster
Shrimp

Goosefoot
Beet and beet sugar
Spinach
Swiss chard

Morning Glory
Sweet potato
Yam

Beech
Chestnut

Parsley
Parsley

Rose
Blackberry
Dewberry
Loganberry
Raspberry
Strawberry
Youngberry

Myrtle
Allspice
Cloves
Guava
Paprika
Pimiento

Ginger
Cardamom
Ginger
Turmeric

Legumes
Alfalfa (sprouts)
Beans: fava, lima, mung, navy, string, kidney, black-eyed peas (cowpea)
Carob, carob syrup
Chickpea (garbanzo)
Fenugreek
Gum acacia
Gum tragacanth
Jicama
Kudzu
Lentil
Licorice
Pea
Peanut, peanut oil
Red clover
Senna: lecithin, soy flour, soy grits, soy milk, soy oil
Tamarind
Tonka bean, coumarin

Gourds
Pumpkin
Squash
Cucumber
Canteloupe
Muskmelon
Honeydew
Persian melon
Casaba
Watermelon

Lily
Aloe
Asparagus
Chive
Garlic
Leek
Onion

Banana
Banana

Pomme
Apple: cider, vinegar, pectin
Pear
Quince, quince seed

Plum
Plum, prune
Cherry
Peach
Apricot
Nectarine
Almond

Laurel
Avocado
Cinnamon
Bay leaves

Potato
Eggplant
Ground cherry
Pepine (melon pear)
Pepper (capsicum): bell (sweet), cayenne, chili, paprika, pimiento
Potato
Tobacco
Tomatillo
Tomato
Tree tomato

Pheasant
Chicken, eggs
Peafowl
Pheasant
Quail
Duck
Turkey
Squab
Goose

Mammals
Pork: ham, bacon

Composite
Leaf lettuce
Head lettuce
Endive
Escarole
Artichoke
Dandelion
Oyster plant
Chicory

Bovine
Beef cattle: beef by-products (gelatin, oleomargarine, rennin [rennet], sausage casings, suet)
Milk products: butter, cheese, ice cream, lactose, spray dried milk, yogurt
Veal
Buffalo
Goat (kid): cheese, milk ice cream
Sheep (domestic): lamb, Rocky Mountain sheep, mutton

Mint
Mint
Peppermint
Spearmint
Thyme
Sage
Marjoram
Savory

Orchid
Vanilla

The following table is an example of food selections based on food families on a four-day rotation diet. For any given day, you can choose any of the foods listed. This table is subdivided into different food groups to assist you with ideas for your menu planning.

ROTATION DIET BY DAY

Group	Day 1	Day 2	Day 3	Day 4
Proteins	Chicken Goose Cornish hen Mackerel Duck Sea bass Eggs	Beef Red snapper Herring Sardines Lamb Veal Pork	Clams Scallops Crab Shrimp Lobster Swordfish Oyster Trout Salmon	Cod Sole Haddock Turkey Hake Tuna Halibut Venison Pike

Vegetables	Broccoli
	Brussels sprouts
	Cabbage
	Cauliflower
	Water chestnut
		Artichokes Olives
		Asparagus Onions
		Garlic Potatoes
		Green peppers Tomatoes
		Lettuce
			Carrots Parsnip
			Celery Pumpkin
			Cucumbers Squash
			Okra Zucchini
				Beets Jicama
				Beans: Peas
				  fava Spinach
				  lima Sprouts
				  mung
				  green beans

Starches	Agar Quinoa Sweet potato	Barley Soy flour Kamut Spelt Millet Teff Oat Wheat Rice	Amaranth Buckwheat Sesame meal	Arrowroot Green beans Mung beans Tapioca
Fruits	Banana Berries Guava Pineapple	Apple Mango Apricot Peach Avocado Pear Cherry Plum Grape Raisin	Kiwi Melons Persimmon Pomegranate Rhubarb	Cranberry Blueberry Lemon Lime Orange
Nuts	Macadamia Pecan Litchi Walnut	Almond Filbert Cashew Hazelnut Chestnut Pistachio	Pine nuts Pumpkin seeds Sesame seeds	Brazil nuts Peanuts Soy nuts
Oils	Canola Flaxseed	Olive Safflower	Cottonseed Sesame	Peanut Soy
Sweeteners	Cocoa Honey Vanilla	Almond syrup Malt syrup Rice syrup	Maple syrup	Carob Coconut
Spices	Basil Sage Oregano Thyme Rosemary	Allspice Cinnamon Bay leaves Cloves	Anise Dill Caraway Fennel Coriander Parsley	Nutmeg Pepper

Dairy	Goat's milk		Cheeses: Cow's milk
			  Cheddar Yogurt
			  Cottage
			  Mozzarella
			  Ricotta
			  Swiss
			  Parmesan	

The following are sample menus for a four-day rotation diet. Other foods can certainly be added if you desire, or omitted if you have been found to be allergic to them.

SAMPLE MENUS FOR A ROTATION DIET

Day 1	Day 2	Day 3	Day 4

Breakfast
2 hard boiled eggs
Fresh strawberries
    and raspberries
Pineapple juice
	Cream of rice with rice
	    milk and raisins
	Grape juice
		Amaranth cereal
		    with milk
		½ cantaloupe
		Herbal tea
			Apples with peanut butter
			Cranberry juice

Snack Banana	Peach	Pumpkin seeds	Orange

Lunch
Quinoa and herbs
Brussels sprouts
Collard greens
	Melted cheese and
	    broiled tomato on
	    spelt bread
		Baked potato
		Poached salmon
		Steamed carrots
		    and celery
			Broiled tuna
			Lentils with soy sauce

Snack Walnuts and pecans	Almonds, cashews, or nectarine	Honeydew melon	Brazil nuts

Dinner
Chicken breast
Baked yam
Steamed cauliflower
    and broccoli
	Beef or veal
	Salad of lettuce,
	    asparagus, tomato, avocado
	Steamed artichoke
	Plum pudding
		Baked swordfish
		Buckwheat groats
		Baked zucchini
		    and squash
		Watermelon
			Turkey breast
			Green beans
			Sprout salad with jicama
			Fresh steamed peas
			Tapioca pudding

Elimination Diet

An elimination diet requires persistence and patience, but may be the surest way to ascertain if a specific food is causing symptoms. When instituting an elimination diet, completely avoid ingesting the foods that are most often the source of food allergies. These foods will then be added back one at a time to see which, if any, are triggering your symptoms. Use the list below as a guideline for initiating an elimination diet.

During the diet, do not eat in restaurants and carefully check the labels of any prepared foods you buy so that you do not eat any eliminated foods inadvertently. Eat acceptable foods in their pure form. Avoid foods such as hot dogs and soft drinks, which contain additives such as preservatives and coloring agents. Take only those medications approved by your physician.

Elimination Diet Suggestions

For one to two weeks, completely avoid the following foods:

1. Beef (including soups and sauces with a beef base)
2. Chicken (including soups and sauces with a chicken base)
3. Chocolate
4. Coffee and tea
5. Corn (including corn meal and corn syrup)
6. Egg ("hidden" in many products, especially baked goods, so check labels carefully)
7. Milk (including cheese, yogurt, ice cream, and baked goods containing milk)
8. Oats
9. Oranges
10. Peanuts
11. Pork (including cold cuts)
12. Potatoes, white
13. Preservatives (such as BHA, BHT, citric acid, and MSG)
14. Soy products
15. Wheat ("hidden" in most baked goods, so check labels carefully)

After the elimination interval, add back one food per day. Keep a diary as to how you feel. If symptoms occur within the first twenty-four hours, it might be an indication that you are sensitive to that particular food. It may be necessary to avoid that food for an extended period of time. Some people find that they feel tired, sluggish, foggy, gassy, swollen, or anxious after eating foods to which they are sensitive, while others may notice a change in their pulse rate or handwriting.

What Foods Can I Eat on an Elimination Diet?

After reading the previous section, you may have thought that there was nothing left to eat. The following table will provide some suggestions for food selections during your elimination diet. Remember to drink several glasses of water per day, preferably spring or filtered.

FOODS PERMITTED ON AN ELIMINATION DIET

Vegetables	Fruits	Meat and Fish	Nuts and Seeds	Sweeteners
Artichokes	Apricots	Clams	Almonds	Clover honey
Asparagus	Bananas	Cornish game hens	Brazil nuts	Date sugar
Avocados	Berries	Crab	Butternuts	Pure maple syrup
Beets	Cantaloupe	Deer	Cashews	
Broccoli	Casaba	Dove	Chestnuts	**Beverages**
Brussels sprouts	Cherries	Duck	Filberts	Juices from allowed
Cabbage	Coconut	Fish	Hazelnuts	fruits diluted
Carrots	Dates	Frog legs	Hickory nuts	with water
Cauliflower	Figs	Goose	Macadamia nuts	Mineral water
Celery	Grapes	Quail	Pecans	Spring water
Collards	Honeydew melon	Lamb	Pistachios	
Cucumbers	Kiwi fruit	Lobster	Pumpkin seeds	**Oils**
Greens	Mango	Oysters	Sesame seeds	Olive oil
Beet	Muskmelon	Pheasant	Sunflower seeds	Safflower oil
Mustard	Nectarines	Rabbit	Tahini	Sesame oil
Turnip	Papaya	Salmon	Walnuts	Sunflower oil
Other	Peaches	Scallops	Water chestnuts	
Jerusalem artichokes	Pears	Shrimp		**Miscellaneous**
Jicama	Persimmons	Squirrel		Bay leaves
Kale	Pineapple	Tuna		Buckwheat groats
Leeks	Plums	Turkey		Caraway
Okra	Pomegranates			Celery seed
Olives	Prunes			Cumin
Parsley	Rhubarb			Dill
Parsnips	Watermelon			Vinegar
Pumpkin				Sea salt
Radishes				
Rutabagas				
Spinach				
Squash				
Acorn				
Butternut				
Pattypan				
Summer				
Sweet potatoes				
Turnips				
Watercress				
Zucchini				

FOODS TO AVOID ON AN ELIMINATION DIET

Cereals
Corn
Cereal mixtures (granola)
Foods containing wheat (most breads and
   baked goods, and pasta)

Beverages
Coffee and creamer
Fruit beverages, except those so specified
Kool-Aid® and powdered drink beverages
Milk or any type of dairy drink with casein
   or whey
Soda pop

Vegetables
Corn
Peas

Meat and Fish
Artificially colored meat
   or hamburger
Bacon
Ham
Hot dogs
Luncheon meats
Smoked salmon

Fruits
Fresh, frozen, or canned citrus

Snacks
Corn chips
Chocolate or anything
   with cocoa
Hard candy
Ice cream or sherbet

Miscellaneous
NutraSweet®
Aspartame®
Saccharin
Cheese
Colored pills or liquid medicines
   (consult doctor first)
Dyed or colored products such as vitamins,
   mouthwash, toothpaste, cough syrup
Eggs
Gelatins and puddings
Jelly or jam
Margarine or diet spreads
   (unless no dyes and corn)
Peanut butter, peanuts
Sorbitol
Sugar, fructose, dextrose

SUGGESTED MENUS FOR AN ELIMINATION DIET

Breakfast
1. Rice cakes with almond butter, prune juice
2. Buckwheat groats with fruit and nuts, pear juice
3. Fruit salad of strawberries, blueberries, raspberries, cold poached salmon

Lunch
1. Baked turkey, salad (spinach or watercress, carrots, radishes, and cucumber) seasoned with sea salt, pear vinegar, and olive oil, steamed cauliflower
2. Shrimp salad (shrimp, celery, parsley, oil, and salt) in avocado, carrot or sweet potato chips, apple
3. Nut butter (almond or cashew, available in health food stores or make your own from any nut)
   or tahini on celery and carrot sticks or pear and banana slices, vegetable soup or salad

Dinner
1. Baked or broiled orange roughy (or similar whitefish), cabbage and carrot slaw with oil, pear
   vinegar, and honey, steamed broccoli
2. Baked turkey, steamed cabbage, baked butternut squash, fresh fruit salad of apples, pears, peaches, and grapes
3. Broiled swordfish with carrots, celery, pineapple, and cashews, steamed asparagus

Snack
1. Avocado dip with celery and carrot sticks
2. Frozen banana with honey and nuts
3. Noncitrus fruit and nuts

Wheat-Free Diet

Many people have been found to be allergic or sensitive to wheat or wheat-containing products. Many foods may contain hidden sources of wheat. Therefore, it is important to read all labels carefully.

FOODS PERMITTED ON A WHEAT-FREE DIET

Breads
Homemade breads, cakes,
    biscuits made from barley, rye,
    oats, and brown rice flour
Millet
Pumpernickel
Rice
Rye
Spelt

Cereals
Amaranth
Corn
Kamut
Oat bran
Rice
Spelt
Teff

Seasonings
Barley miso
Fresh and dried herbs
Pepper
Sea salt
Sesame salt
Tamari
Yeast extracts

Pastas
Buckwheat
Corn
Quinoa
Rice

Snacks
Carrot chips
Corn chips
Oat cakes
Popcorn
Potato chips
Rice cakes
Rice chips
Taro chips
Wheat-free cookies
Wheat-free crackers

Miscellaneous
All animal products
Arrowroot
Barley flour
Beans, lentils, and peas
Fresh fruit salad
Kudzu
Potato flour
Sea vegetables
Soy flour
Vegetables

FOODS TO AVOID ON A WHEAT-FREE DIET

Breads*
Biscuits
Bran
Buns
Cakes
Cookies
Crackers
Doughnuts
Matzoh
Non-rye crispbreads
Pancakes
Pastries
Rolls
Scones
Wheat germ

Snacks
Chocolates and other sweets
Instant coffees
Malted milks
Puddings containing semolina or
    refined flour

Seasonings
Monosodium glutamate (MSG)

Cereals
All cereals containing wheat,
    wheat germ, or bran

Miscellaneous
Alcoholic beverages
Battered and breaded foods
Bulgur, couscous
Bologna
Bouillon cubes
Dumplings
Processed meats,
    corned beef, sausages,
    beef burgers, hamburgers
Processed cheeses and spreads
Spaghetti, macaroni, pastas
Thickeners in soups, stews,
    and gravies (corn flour)

*If these products are wheat-free, they are permitted.

Are There Alternatives to Wheat?

If you are sensitive to wheat, there are many other flours now available that can be used as a wheat substitute. Many brands of breads and cakes are already made with wheat-free products. Be sure to read labels at your favorite health food store to determine which products are suitable for you. For those who want to bake with wheat-free flour, the following are excellent substitutes for wheat flour.

I have found that many of my patients feel healthier on a wheat-free diet. Many have been able to shed undesirable and difficult-to-lose pounds, feel an increase in energy, and notice that their mind is clearer. Others have reported that their intestinal gas and bloating subsides and intestinal swelling is reduced. I have also seen that a wheat-free diet may help in some cases of attention-deficit disorder and autism.

WHEAT FLOUR SUBSTITUTES Each of the substitutions equals 1 cup of wheat flour.

Amaranth flour	⅞ cup, lighter baked goods can be made by substituting ¼ to ¾ parts flour with brown rice, oats, soy, arrowroot, tapioca, or potato flour. Good for breading.
Arrowroot flour	¾ cup or ½ cup arrowroot plus ½ cup of another flour or nut meal adds flavor and nutritional value to pancakes and baked goods. Great as a thickening agent.
Barley flour	1¼ cup, very good in pancakes and baked goods, but closely related to wheat in allergenic properties.
Brown rice flour	⅞ cup, or ½ brown rice flour and ½ oat flour in cookies and pie crusts.
Buckwheat flour	¾ cup, good in pancakes, baked goods, and breading. Kasha can be ground into buckwheat flour.
Cassava flour	¾ cup, good in baked goods and as a thickening agent.
Chickpea flour	¾ cup, good in flat breads, cookies, and as a thickening agent.
Jerusalem artichoke flour	¾ to ⅝ cup, good for baked goods.
Malanga flour	¾ cup, good for baked goods, dumplings, and as a thickener.
Spelt flour	⅔ cup, good for baked goods. Since it is generally heavier than wheat flour, you may also want to add ⅓ cup of potato or rice flour.

Gluten-Free Diet

Does Gluten in Whole Wheat Bread Cause Abdominal Bloating?

Gluten is a protein substance found in cereal grains such as wheat, barley, rye, and oats. Gluten sensitivity is very common and can lead to a variety of symptoms. Finding out whether or not you are gluten intolerant usually takes some investigation by your physician. This can be diagnosed by either allergy skin testing, or blood or urine studies.

SYMPTOMS OF GLUTEN SENSITIVITY INCLUDE:

- Bloating
- Cramping
- Colitis
- Diarrhea
- Gas
- Hair loss

GLUTEN MAY ALSO BE A FACTOR IN:

- Autism
- Arthritis
- Schizophrenia
- Multiple sclerosis

Treatment for Gluten Intolerance

If you are gluten intolerant, avoiding it is the mainstay of treatment. Even small amounts of gluten may cause symptoms. I have seen many patients who have had a long history of Crohn's disease, ulcerative colitis, or intestinal gas, bloating, and cramping who improve greatly once they have removed the gluten from their diet. Check all labels for hidden gluten ingredients. The following list will provide you with choices on a gluten-free diet.

FOODS PERMITTED ON A GLUTEN-FREE DIET

Meat
Fish
Poultry
Cheese
Fresh vegetables
Fresh fruit
Breads and cereals made from permitted flours
Eggs
Milk
Fruit juices

Tea and herbal teas
Coffee
Flours and thickening agents:
  Arrowroot starch
  Corn flour, corn starch, corn meal
  Potato flour, potato starch flour
  Rice bran
  Rice flours: plain, brown, sweet
  Soy flour
  Tapioca starch

FOODS TO AVOID ON A GLUTEN-FREE DIET (cont.)

Wheat, barley, rye, oats, millet, buckwheat, bulgur, kasha

Pasta, cereals, and bakery products made from the above grains

Processed food with hidden gluten such as frankfurters, sausage, cold cuts, soups, and baked beans

Coffee substitutes made with cereal

Milk drinks mixed with malt

Beer or ale

Dairy-Free Diet

Are There Alternatives to Dairy Products?

Many people are intolerant to dairy products because they lack the enzyme lactase, which is necessary to break down lactose, or milk sugar. It has been estimated that nearly fifty million Americans suffer from lactose intolerance, which is more prevalent among certain ethnic groups. Nearly 90 percent of all Asian Americans and 75 percent of African Americans, Jews, Native Americans, and Hispanics have insufficient levels of the enzyme lactase needed to properly digest dairy products. Common symptoms associated with lactose intolerance and milk or dairy sensitivity include intestinal gas, bloating, indigestion, cramping, foul-smelling stools, fat in the stool, diarrhea, or even constipation.

Even if you are lactose intolerant, it may still be possible to enjoy dairy products without experiencing abdominal discomfort. You may find that a natural dairy digestive supplement, such as Lactaid caplets or drops, make dairy products easier to digest. Lactaid milk, which is lactose-reduced milk, is also well-tolerated by many people who are sensitive to regular milk.

Lactase is normally manufactured in the small intestine and is usually produced in sufficient quantities during infancy and childhood. However, in some people, the production of lactase decreases as they grow older, making them more prone to lactose intolerance. Be aware that lactose is also used as an inactive ingredient in more than 20 percent of prescription drugs and about 6 percent of the over-the-counter medications. If you are extremely lactose intolerant, it's always best to read medication labels.

If you suspect that dairy products may be contributing to your symptoms, try eliminating milk and related products from your diet for seven to ten days and then reintroduce them. If your symptoms recur, there is a high probability that you will do better to avoid dairy products. If you are concerned about consuming adequate amounts of calcium while following a dairy-free diet, remember to increase your intake of the foods discussed on page 108.

HIDDEN DAIRY MAY BE IN THESE FOODS

Au gratin foods	Candies	Doughnuts	Pancakes	Soda cracker
Bavarian cream	Cheeses	Flour mixes	Pie crust	Soufflé
Biscuits	Chowders	Fritters	Salad dressing	Soups (creamed)
Breads	Cocoa drinks	Gravies	Scalloped dishes	Spumoni
Buttermilk	Creamed foods			Waffles
Cakes	Curds			Whey yogurt
Cookies	Custards			

DAIRY-FREE ALTERNATIVES

Milk

Soy milk	Oat milk
Rice milk	Almond milk
Goat milk	

Ice Cream

Sorbet
Rice-based ice cream
Soybean ice cream

Cheese

Soy cheese
Goat cheese
Almond cheese

Hypoglycemia

Hypoglycemia is characterized by the inability to effectively metabolize glucose and carbohydrates. With hypoglycemia, your blood sugar may fall to an abnormally low level. This can be differentiated from hyperglycemia, or diabetes, which is characterized by an elevated glucose level. Hypoglycemia is frequently accompanied by excess insulin secretion from your pancreas, which will in turn drive your blood sugar level to an abnormally low range. It may be necessary to follow a hypoglycemic diet (as discussed on pages 110 and 111) to help regulate your blood sugar.

The condition known as reactive hypoglycemia occurs when your blood sugar level drops a few hours after eating a particular meal, frequently one that is laden with sugar or processed foods. In this case, your blood sugar may initially rise beyond the normal range, only to be driven down to below normal levels once your pancreas secretes insulin in its effort to metabolize the food.

Another form of reactive hypoglycemia can occur if you have skipped meals or avoided food intake for a prolonged period of time. In this example, your body does not have enough fuel to maintain blood sugar in its normal range.

Reactive hypoglycemia can be diagnosed by having your doctor request a five- or six-hour *glucose tolerance test*. In this case, you will be given a carbohydrate solution to drink and your blood sugar level will be assessed each hour.

In a typical reactive hypoglycemic pattern, the blood sugar level will initially rise, perhaps beyond the higher limits of normal and then fall precipitously into a below-normal range. When I am concerned about diagnosing reactive hypoglycemia, I frequently prescribe a *glucose insulin tolerance test*. This laboratory study not only assesses your glucose level but also measures the insulin output. If your insulin levels are elevated, especially during the first three hours of testing, you might be at a higher risk for developing reactive hypoglycemia or even diabetes at some time in the future. If you are found to have reactive hypoglycemia, try to go no longer than three hours without eating.

COMMON SYMPTOMS OF HYPOGLYCEMIA

- Headaches
- Anxiety
- Panic attacks
- Dizziness
- Light-headedness
- Jittery feelings
- Irritability
- Fainting/blackouts
- Forgetfulness
- Heart palpitations
- Mood swings
- Drowsiness

There are two main schools of thought regarding treatment for this medical condition. The first advocates a high-carbohydrate diet, while the second promotes a high-protein diet. I generally recommend a high-complex-carbohydrate diet initially for patients suffering from hypoglycemia. If you have not noted any improvement in your symptoms after three months of following the diet, you might then want to change to a high-protein diet with moderate amounts of carbohydrates.

Choosing your approach may depend on your specific body type and your body's response to sugar. Both diets stress the total elimination of refined sugar, refined carbohydrates, refined flour, and processed foods. In addition to a proper diet, nutritional supplements may be helpful in normalizing your blood sugar response, reducing your symptoms of hypoglycemia. Specifically, I have found that vitamin C, B complex, vitamin E, and the minerals chromium, magnesium, manganese, and zinc can all play a vital role in assisting with blood sugar metabolism.

FOODS RECOMMENDED FOR A HYPOGLYCEMIC DIET

Protein: An adequate amount of protein must be ingested each day. This can be obtained from nuts and seeds, and beans and grains as well as fish, cheese, eggs, chicken, turkey, and red meat.

Fruits		Vegetables			Grains and Beans	Miscellaneous
Apples	*Limit:*	Alfalfa sprouts*	Jerusalem	Spinach	Adzuki beans	Carob chips and
Apricots	Dried fruit	Artichoke*	artichoke	Sprouts	Amaranth	carob powder
Blackberries	Avocado	Asparagus*	Jicama*	Squash	Barley	Corn meal
Blueberries	Bananas	Bamboo shoots	Kale	summer and	Buckwheat	Cornstarch for
Cantaloupe	Cherries	Bean sprouts*	Kohlrabi*	winter	Bulgur	thickening
Cranberries	Coconut,	Beans	Leeks	String beans*	Corn	Cracked wheat
Currants	unsweetened**	Beet greens*	Lettuce	Summer squash	Couscous	Decaf coffee
Gooseberries	Dates	Beets	Lima beans	Sweet potatoes	Garbanzo beans	Egg whites
Grapefruit	Figs	Broccoli*	Mushrooms*	Tomatoes	Lentils	Ground raisins for
Honeydew	Grapes	Brussels sprouts*	Mustard greens	Turnips*	Millet	cooking
Huckleberries	Maraschino	Cabbage	Okra	Water chestnuts	Mung beans	Jerusalem artichoke
Kumquat	cherries	Carrots	Onions*	Watercress	Navy beans	flour
Lemons	Olives**	Cauliflower*	Parsley	Zucchini squash*	Oats	Molasses for cooking
Limes	Persimmons	Celery	Peas		Peas	Non-fat milk
Loganberries	Prune juice	Celery root	Pickles		Pinto beans	Non-fat yogurt
Mulberries	Prunes	Chicory	Potatoes		Quinoa	Nuts and seeds**
Muskmelon		Chives	Pumpkin*		Rice	Oat flour
Nectarines		Collard	Radishes*		Rye	Oatmeal
Oranges		Cucumber*	Red peppers*		Sorghum wheat	Oils: canola, olive,
Papaya		Dandelion greens	Rhubarb*		Soybeans	flaxseed
Peaches		Eggplant*	Rutabaga		Tempeh	Soy flour
Pears		Endive	Sauerkraut*		Tofu	Unflavored gelatin
Pineapples		Escarole	Scallions*		Yeast	(flavor w/juice,
Quince		Garlic	Shallots*			not water)
Raspberries		Gingerroot	Soybeans			Wheat flour
Strawberries		Green peppers	Spaghetti squash*			Whole wheat products
Tangerines						Whole wheat cereal
Watermelon						

* Highly recommended due to low carbohydrate content.
** Limit due to high carbohydrate content.

TIP

- Exercise regularly to normalize glucose metabolism.
- Watch out for rancid oil, nuts, and seeds.
- Avoid caffeine, nicotine, and alcohol.

- Eat small meals 5–6 times a day.
- Do not skip meals.
- Avoid stress. It aggravates hypoglycemia.

FOODS TO AVOID ON A HYPOGLYCEMIC DIET

Most of the foods listed below are not permitted because of their high carbohydrate (sugar and starch) content. Refined carbohydrates (white sugar and white flour products) are especially poor food choices because they provide energy (calories) with very little nutrition (vitamins, minerals, and protein) essential for good body function and repair. By eliminating these foods, you can also take a major step towards maintaining your ideal body weight. Most of these foods provide so-called "empty calories." Generally, both underweight and overweight individuals benefit from this basic diet.

General		Sugars	Bread and Grains	Beverages
Apple butter	Ice cream	*Sugar listed on labels may be termed:*	Biscuits	Artificial fruit drinks
Brown sugar	Icing		Croutons	Beer
Brownies	Jam		Enriched white bread	Chocolate milk
Cakes	Jellies	Corn sweeteners	Flour tortillas	Cocktails
Candies	Luncheon meats	Dextrose	Graham crackers	Cocoa
Candy-coated fruits	Maple syrup	Fructose	Macaroni	Coffee
Candy-coated nuts	Marmalade	Galactose	Muffins	Cordials
Chocolate syrup	Marshmallows	Maltose	Noodles	Drinks containing
Cocoa	Pastries	Sucrose	Pancakes	white sugar
Corn syrup	Pies		Pretzels	Grape juice
Custard	Powdered sugar	*Hidden sugars may be found in:*	Rolls	Instant breakfast drinks
Doughnuts	Pudding		Saltines	Malts
Flavored gelatin	Sugared peanut butter	Barbeque sauce	Soda crackers	Milk shakes
Fruit packed in syrup	White flour	Bottled salad dressing	Spaghetti	Soft drinks
Glazes	White sugar	Chili sauce	Sugar-coated cereals	Sweetened fruit juices
		Cranberry sauce	Waffles	Wine
		Ketchup		
		Mustard sauce		
		Steak sauce		

SAMPLE MENU FOR A HYPOGLYCEMIC DIET

Upon arising	4 oz grapefruit juice
Breakfast	1 slice cantaloupe, 1 fried egg, 1 slice whole wheat toast with butter
Midmorning	4 oz tomato juice
Lunch	Salad with tomato, cucumber, and red pepper, broiled breast of chicken or brown rice with lentils, string beans
Midafternoon	1 orange, pumpkin seeds, hummous
Half-hour before dinner	4 oz vegetable juice
Dinner	Homemade soup, salad, broiled fish or stir-fried tofu over couscous, baked potato, broccoli, fresh fruit cup for dessert
Evening snack	Celery and carrot sticks with cream cheese dip or natural peanut butter

Weight-Loss Diet

It has been estimated that over 50 percent of the American adult population is overweight. Recently the number of overweight children and teenagers has also increased. There are many weight-loss plans that may be successful, depending on your individual body type and biochemistry. You may find that a moderate- or high-protein diet is best while others prefer a low-fat, high-complex-carbohydrate diet, as shown below. Regardless of the plan you follow, avoid sugar and refined carbohydrates as much as possible.

SUGGESTED MENUS	EXAMPLES
Breakfast	
2 oz fresh fruit juice	2 oz orange juice
1 cup whole grain cereal	1 cup oatmeal
Snack	
1 fruit	1 apple
Lunch	
3 oz protein	3 oz broiled fish or chicken or
$\frac{1}{2}$ cup whole grain	$\frac{1}{2}$ cup brown rice or millet
$\frac{1}{2}$ cup beans or lentils	$\frac{1}{2}$ cup black beans
1 cup vegetables	Steamed broccoli and cauliflower
Salad with 2 tbsp dressing	Lettuce, tomato, cucumber salad with
	flaxseed oil, lemon, onion, garlic, and herb dressing
Snack	
Vegetable juice or crudités	Celery and carrot sticks
Dinner	
3 oz protein or	3 oz broiled fish with lemon
$\frac{1}{2}$ cup beans or lentils	$\frac{1}{2}$ cup couscous
$\frac{1}{2}$ cup whole grain	$\frac{1}{2}$ cup lentils
1 cup vegetables	1 small baked potato topped with dressing of
	mustard, chopped fresh garlic, chopped tomato
Salad with 2 tbsp dressing	Endive, onion, radishes
	Dressing: fresh-squeezed lemon juice, garlic, and pumpkin
	and sesame seed dressing
Snack	
Low-fat snack	1 cup air-popped popcorn or rice cake with apple butter
Vegetables	Red pepper strips
Fruit	Peach

Headache Sufferers' Diet

Many of you may be troubled by chronic headaches. Did you know that headaches are frequently caused by food allergies or sensitivities? As a result, it may be necessary to change your food selections to help reduce the frequency, severity, and duration of your headaches. You may find that food preservatives, additives, and colorings can trigger headaches. Sugar and artificial sweeteners can also provoke headaches. Be sure to read labels to avoid ingesting "hidden" substances. Eating at regular intervals to prevent blood sugar fluctuations may also benefit headache sufferers. Waking up at the same time every day, even on weekends, may also prevent blood sugar fluctuations and the resulting headaches. Try to avoid the following foods if you suffer from headaches.

FOODS TO AVOID FOR HEADACHE SUFFERERS

Dairy	Meat and Fish	Fruits and Vegetables
Milk	Chicken livers	Avocados
Egg	Fermented sausage	Bananas (no more than 1/2 per day)
Ripened cheese:	Bologna	Canned figs
Brie	Salami	Citrus fruits (no more than 1 orange
Camembert	Pepperoni	per day)
Cheddar	Hot dogs	Corn
Emmentaler	Pork	Fermented, pickled, or
Gruyère	(no more than 2–3	marinated foods
Stilton	times per week)	Peanut butter
Sour cream	Herring	Onions
Yogurt		Pods or broad beans
		Lima
		Navy
		Pea pods
		Seeds
		Sunflower
		Sesame
		Pumpkin

Beverages	Additives	Other Foods
All alcoholic beverages	Artificial sweeteners,	Breads and baked goods
Tea	Aspartame products such as:	Chinese foods
Coffee	Equal	Pizza
Cola beverages	NutraSweet	Soybeans
	Spoonful	Vinegar
	Benzoic acid	
	Caffeine	
	Ethanol	
	Monosodium glutamate (MSG)	
	Phenylethylamine	
	Processed foods, soups, and	
	TV dinners	
	Salt/sodium	
	Sodium metabisulfite	
	Sodium nitrate	
	Theobromine	
	Tyramine	

Feingold's Low Salicylate Diet

Could Your Hyperactive Child Benefit from a Low-Salicylate Diet?

In the 1970s, pediatrician Benjamin Feingold, M.D., recommended the exclusion of salicylates, substances found in artificial colors and flavors as well as many foods, from the diet of hyperactive children. Dr. Feingold found that salicylates may be responsible for hyperactivity and learning disabilities in children. Even today, many parents find that this diet is successful in reducing their children's symptoms of hyperactivity. Use the following table as a rough guide to refining your child's diet.

SALICYLATE CONTENT OF VARIOUS FOODS

	Very High	High	Moderate	Low	Very Low	None

Fruits (fresh unless otherwise noted)	Apricots
	Berries (canned)
	  Black
	  Blue
	  Boysen
	  Cran
	  Logan
	Berries (fresh)
	  Raspberries
	  Strawberries
	Currants,
	  Fresh or dried
	Guava, canned
	Oranges
	Raisins
	Pineapple, fresh
	  or canned
	Prunes, canned
		Sweet cherry
		Grape, most
		  varieties
		Mulberry
		Tangelo
			Apples:
			  Granny Smith
			Avocados
			Figs:
			  Calanda, dried
			Grapefruit
			Oranges, mandarin
			Nectarines
			Peaches
				Apple:
				  Red delicious
				  Jonathan
				Figs
				Kiwi fruit
				Lemon
				Loquat
				Lychee, canned
				Pears with skin
				Persimmon
				Pineapple
				  juice
				Plums
				Watermelon
					Apple:
					  Golden
					  delicious
					Mango
					Passion fruit
					Plums:
					  Kelsey
					  Wilson
					Pomegranate
					Rhubarb
					Tamarillo
						Bananas
						Pears

Vegetables (fresh unless otherwise noted)	Pickles
	Endive
	Green olives
	Pepper:
	  Red chili
	  Sweet
	  Green
	Radish
	Tomato sauce,
	  canned
		Broad beans
		Fava, dried
		Chicory
		Cucumbers
		Eggplant
		Watercress
		Zucchini
			Alfalfa
			Broccoli
			Okra, canned
			Peppers:
			  green
			  chili
			  yellow
			  green chili
			Spinach
			Baby squash
			Tomato soup
			Tomato paste
				Beetroot
				Carrots
				Cauliflower
				Eggplant,
				  peeled
				Parsnips
				Horseradish
				Mushrooms
				Black olives
				Sweet potato
				Onion
				Spinach,
				  frozen
				Tomato juice
				Turnip
					Asparagus
					Green beans
					Bean sprouts
					Red cabbage
					Chives
					Leeks
					Peas, dried:
					  yellow split
					Pimientos,
					  canned
					Potato,
					  white with
					  skins
					Pumpkin
					Shallots
					Sweet corn
					Tomatoes
						Bamboo shoots
						Beans, dried:
						  black-eyed
						  soy
						  lima
						  mung
						Green cabbage
						Celery
						Chickpeas
						Lentils, red, brown
						Lettuce
						Peas, dried:
						  green split
						Potato, white
						  without skin

	Very High	High	Moderate	Low	Very Low	None
Cereal Grains	— — — — — — —	— — — — — — —	— — — — — — —	— — — — — — —	— — — — — — —	Arrowroot powder Barley Buckwheat Millet Oats Rice Rye Wheat
Protein Foods	— — — — — — — — —	— — — — — — — — —	— — — — — — — — —	— — — — — — — — —	Liver Prawns Scallops	Beef Chicken Eggs Kidney Lamb Oysters Pork Salmon, canned Tripe Tuna, canned Milk
Dairy	— — — —	— — — —	— — — —	— — — —	Camembert Mozzarella Blue cheese	Cream Yogurt Cottage cheese Cheddar cheese
Nuts and Seeds	Almonds Water chestnuts, canned	Peanuts, unskinned	Macadamia Pine nuts Pistachio	Brazil nuts Coconut, dry Peanut butter Sesame seed Walnuts	Cashew Hazelnuts Pecans Sunflower seeds	Poppyseed
Sugars and Candies	Honey Licorice Some mints	Lifesavers, peppermint	— — — — —	Molasses	Golden syrup	Carob powder Cocoa powder Maple syrup White sugar, granulated
Beverages	Tetley tea bags Twinings teas	Maxwell House instant coffee Peppermint tea	Nescafé instant coffee	Coca-Cola Herb tea, fruit Herb tea, rosehip	Herb tea, chamomile	Nescafé decaffeinated coffee
Alcoholic Beverages	Benedictine Drambuie Port	Tia Maria Rum Some wines	Cointreau Sherry Some wines	Beers Hard apple cider Hennessey brandy Some wines	— — — — —	Gilbey's gin Smirnoff vodka Johnnie Walker whiskey

	Very High	High	Moderate	Low	Very Low	None
Herbs and Spices (dry powders only)	Curry Hot paprika Thyme	Dill Turmeric	Garam masala Oregano Rosemary	Aniseed Canella Cayenne Cinnamon Five spice Mace Mustard powder Sage Tarragon	Allspice Bay leaf Basil Cardamom Caraway Celery Chili powder Cloves Fennel Fenugreek Nutmeg Sweet paprika Pepper, black or white Pimiento powder	Saffron Tandori
Condiments (fresh or liquid)	Worcestershire sauce	Dill, fresh Mint, fresh Ginger, fresh	Vanilla extract White vinegar	Tabasco sauce	Coriander, fresh Garlic, fresh Parsley, fresh	Malt vinegar Soy sauce

Source: Adapted from "Salicylates in Foods," Swain, Dutton, and Truswell, *Journal of the American Dietetic Association.*

Here is a sample of a five-day low salicylate diet. Feel free to make your own diet plan as well.

	Monday	Tuesday	Wednesday	Thursday	Friday
Breakfast	Buckwheat cereal, banana	Oat cereal	Rice cereal	Rye cereal, pecans	Eggs
Snack	Sunflower seeds	Pear	Plum	Kiwi	Golden Delicious apple
Lunch	Tuna on rye, carrots	Grilled eggplant, cauliflower	Cashew butter on wheat	Cottage cheese, figs, pineapple	Yogurt Watermelon
Snack	Mango	Kiwi	Walnuts	Celery	Cashews
Dinner	Lamb, steamed cabbage, lima beans, corn	Lentils, peas, lettuce salad, sweet potato	Salmon, leeks, asparagus	Chicken, white potato, spinach	Beef, green beans, tomatoes, mushrooms

Low-Oxalate Diet
Could Your Diet Be Contributing to Kidney Stones?

Some people have difficulty metabolizing foods that contain oxalate. Oxalic acid can accumulate and contribute to kidney stones. A low-oxalate diet can be effective in reducing the risk of developing calcium oxalate kidney stones, the most common type of kidney stones. If you suspect problems with kidney stones, use the following guidelines to help you reduce oxalate levels. I do not believe that you have to significantly curtail your intake of calcium-containing foods if you are troubled with kidney stones. In fact, some studies have indicated that avoiding calcium-containing foods may have a detrimental affect and trigger the formation of more kidney stones. If you suffer from kidney stones, increase your intake of water as well as foods rich in vitamin B_6 and magnesium, which you can find listed on pages 7 and 10, respectively.

FOODS PERMITTED ON A LOW OXALATE CONTENT

Vegetables	Fruits	Beverages	Miscellaneous
Broccoli	Avocado	Apple juice	Butter
Brussels sprouts	Cherries	Barley water	Cheese, cheddar
Cabbage	Grapes	Cider	Chicken noodle soup
Cauliflower	Mangos	Grapefruit juice	Cornflakes
Chives	Melons	Lemonade	Eggs
Cucumber	Nectarines	Milk	Egg noodles (chow mein)
Lettuce	Peaches	Orange juice	Fish (except sardines)
Mushrooms	Pineapple	Pineapple juice	Jelly
Onions	Plums		Lemon juice
Peas			Lime juice
Potatoes			Macaroni
Radishes			Margarine
Rice			Meats
Turnips			Oatmeal
			Poultry
			Red plum jam

FOODS TO AVOID DUE TO HIGH OXALATE CONTENT

Vegetables	Fruits	Beverages	Miscellaneous
Beans in tomato sauce	Bananas	Decaffeinated	Chocolate
Beets	Berries:	Coffee	Cocoa
Celery	Blackberries	Soda	Corned beef
Collards	Blueberries	Tea	Frozen foods
Dandelion greens	Raspberries		Grits (white corn)
Eggplant	Currants		Peanuts
Escarole	Grapes:		Pecans
Leek	Concord		Preservatives
Okra	Green Goose		Processed lunch
Parsley	Red		meats
Pepper, green	Lemon peel		Soybean crackers
Potatoes, sweet	Lime peel		Wheat germ
Rutabagas	Rhubarb		
Sorrel	Tomatoes		
Spinach			
Summer squash			
Swiss chard			

Anti-Gout Diet

Could Your Joint Pain Be Due to Anchovies in Your Caesar Salad?

Gout is a disease in which uric acid, a breakdown product of purines, builds up in the blood and tissues, resulting in acute inflammatory joint pain or gouty arthritis. This form of arthritis develops in response to the uric acid crystals, which deposit in the synovial fluid of the joints. An attack of gout can be quite painful and is frequently treated with long-term medications. Furthermore, patients with chronic gout are also at risk for kidney disease and uric acid kidney stones.

The first line of defense should be to follow a low-purine diet and to minimize your intake of high-purine foods, especially red meat. As you can see, the highest levels of purines are generally found in animal organ meats and to a lesser degree in legumes and specific beans.

The following table provides guidelines for selecting low-purine foods:

PURINE CONTENT OF FOODS

Foods Highest in Purines 150–825 mg per 100 g	Foods High in Purines 50–150 mg per 100 g	Foods Lowest in Purines 0–15 mg per 100 g
Anchovies	Meat	Fruits—all kinds
Sweetbreads	Poultry	Vegetables—except listed at left
Sardines, in oil	Fish	Most breads
Liver, calf, beef	Lobster	Cereals
Kidneys, beef	Crab	Milk
Meat extracts	Oysters	Eggs
Gravies	Meat soups and broth	All nuts
	Beans, dried	Gelatin
	Peas, dried	Cream soups
	Lentils, dried	
	Spinach	
	Oatmeal	
	Wheat germ and bran	
	Mushrooms	
	Lima beans	
	Navy beans	
	Kidney beans	
	Asparagus	

Glycemic Index and Blood Sugar

Is Your Diet Contributing to Elevated Blood Sugar?

Not all foods elevate blood sugar levels at the same rate. As it turns out, carbohydrate-containing foods can produce a wide range of responses to blood sugar. For example, eating a potato may increase your blood sugar response more than the consumption of an apple. The *glycemic index* indicates the rate at which different carbohydrates break down to produce sugar in your bloodstream. Foods with a high glycemic index are metabolized quickly into sugar, while low-glycemic-index foods generally release sugar into the bloodstream more slowly. High-glycemic-index foods can, in turn, trigger excessive insulin release, which has been associated with diabetes, hypertension, and cardiovascular disease.

If you are diabetic, hypoglycemic, or obese, try to choose foods with a lower glycemic index. The glycemic index for most green vegetables is less than 15. However, the glycemic index is simply one of the many guidelines you should use in making your food selections. Keep an eye on the fat content as well since, for example, high-fat ice cream has a lower glycemic index than a healthier, high-glycemic-index carrot. If you choose to eat high-glycemic-index foods, mix them with healthy fats, protein, and low-glycemic-index foods as well.

In the table below, all listed foods are compared to the effect of ingesting glucose, which has a glycemic index value of 100.

THE GLYCEMIC INDEX OF COMMON FOODS

Grains and Cereal Products

Buckwheat	51
Bread (wheat)	69
Bread (whole grain)	72
Corn	59
Millet	71
Oatmeal	49
Rice (brown)	66
Rice (white)	72
Spaghetti (whole grain)	42
Spaghetti (white)	50

Vegetables

Carrots	92
Parsnips	97
Potato (Red Bliss)	70
Potato (sweet)	48
Yam	51

Dried Legumes

Beans (baked)	40
Beans (green)	31
Beans (kidney)	29
Beans (soy)	15

Lentils	29
Peas (black-eyed)	33
Peas (chick)	36

Fruit

Apples	39
Banana	62
Oranges	40
Orange juice	46
Raisins	64

Sugars

Fructose	20
Glucose	100
Honey	87
Maltose	105
Sucrose	59

Dairy Products

Ice cream	36
Milk (skim)	32
Milk (whole)	34
Yogurt	36

CHAPTER 9

Candida: Yeast-Related Illness

Candida albicans, or candida, is a naturally occurring yeast that is normally held in balance by your body's friendly bacteria.

Unfortunately, this friendly bacteria can be destroyed through the overuse of antibiotics, birth control pills, hormonal changes, a sugar-rich diet, steroids (cortisone and prednisone), or prolonged or acute exposure to chemicals, pesticides, or molds.

When this beneficial bacteria is destroyed, yeasts can proliferate and colonize your body's tissues. This can give rise to a variety of medical complications. The condition is known as candidiasis, the yeast syndrome, or yeast-related illness.

Are Your Headaches Caused by Yeast Overgrowth?

Yeast overgrowth can cause a breakdown in your immune system and a weakening of your immune response. While women seem to be affected more frequently, both men and children are also susceptible to the yeast syndrome. Because candidiasis is not a commonly recognized condition, the failure to identify and treat this syndrome may result in costly medical treatments and unnecessary suffering.

SYMPTOMS ASSOCIATED WITH YEAST OVERGROWTH

Genitourinary	Gastrointestinal	Allergic	Cerebral-Neurological
Chronic vaginal infections	Intestinal bloating/gas	Asthma	Headaches
Menstrual cramps	Intestinal cramps	Hay fever	Depression
PMS	Intestinal mucus	Earaches	Irritability
Chronic urinary tract infections	Irritable bowel syndrome	Hives	Memory lapses
	Diarrhea	Food allergy	Inability to concentrate or brain fog
	Constipation	Chemical sensitivities	

Diagnosis

There is no single diagnostic test to conclusively identify candida yeast overgrowth. A detailed medical history, combined with a therapeutic trial of diet, antifungal supplements, herbs, and medications, can play an important diagnostic role. The medical history should focus on the patient's use of medications, especially antibiotics and birth control pills, as well as the patient's cravings for sweets, refined carbohydates, and alcohol.

Methods of diagnosis also include:
- Score on candida questionnaire
- Allergy skin testing (for candida and yeast sensitivities)

Laboratory testing:
- *through blood work* (measures candida-specific antibodies and/or candida immune complexes)
- *through stool testing* (measures an overgrowth of candida and related yeasts)
- *through cultures* (cultures from other mucous membranes for Candida albicans)

Treatments

In order to treat *Candida albicans* effectively, it is important to treat the whole person. The most effective treatment includes the thorough assessment of the patient's biochemical status, including environmental and nutritional factors.

Before beginning antifungal medication, a review of the following is advisable: food allergies, nutrient imbalances, diet, chemical sensitivities.

Treatment modalities include:

- A dietary program
- Controlling environmental molds and mold spores
- Antifungal medications
- Nutritional supplements
- Allergy desensitization
- Herbs, botanicals, and homeopathics

What Foods May I Eat?

If you are suffering from candida overgrowth or yeast-related illness, eating a diet low in sugar, refined carbohydrates, refined fruit, and yeast-containing foods is perhaps the first step in solving your problem. Some people have to be stricter than others during the initial few weeks. The following foods are generally permitted on an anti-candida diet:

Permitted Food Selections: An Anticandida Diet

Beans and Lentils*

Adzuki	Lentils	Lima beans	Soybeans
Garbanzo beans	Kidney	Navy	

Beverages

Herbal teas	Fresh squeezed juice (Vegetable)	Soy milk, rice milk, goat Milk, coconut milk	Water/seltzer

Fresh Fruits (use sparingly, and if symptoms occur, discontinue use)

Apples	Blueberries	Nectarines	Pineapple
Apricots	Cherries	Oranges	Plums
Avocados	Grapefruit	Papayas	Raspberries
Bananas	Grapes	Peaches	Strawberries
Blackberries	Mangos	Pears	

Grains

Amaranth	Couscous	Oats	Teff
Barley	Corn	Quinoa	Wheat
Brown rice	Millet	Rye	Wild rice
Buckwheat			

Nuts and Seeds (be cautious of stale and moldy nuts)

Almonds	Filberts	Pumpkin seeds	Sunflower seeds
Brazil nuts	Pecans	Sesame seeds	Walnuts
Cashews	Pine nuts		

Oils (use only unprocessed, cold-pressed oils)

Almond	Canola (rape seed)	Linseed	Soy
Apricot kernel	Corn	Olive	Sesame
Avocado	Flax	Safflower	Sunflower
			Walnut

Protein

Beef	Fish (all kinds)	Oysters	Shrimp
Chicken	Game birds	Pheasant	Squirrel
Clams	Goose	Pork	Tofu
Crab	Lamb	Quail	Turkey
Duck	Lobster	Rabbit	Veal
Eggs			

Vegetables

Artichokes	Cauliflower	Kale	Potatoes: red, white*
Asparagus	Celery	Lettuce	Radishes
Beet greens	Collard greens	Mustard greens	Sea vegetables
Beets*	Corn*	Okra	Spinach
Broccoli	Cucumber	Onion	Squash
Brussels sprouts	Eggplant	Parsley	Sweet potatoes*
Cabbage	Green beans	Parsnips	Swiss chard
Carrots*	Green pepper	Peas: green, split*	Tomatoes
			Zucchini

Miscellaneous

Rice cakes	Yeast-free bread, muffins,	Crackers	Seaweed – dulce, kelp,
		Yogurt	arame, wakame, hijiki

*Eat cautiously.

What Foods Should I Avoid?

When selecting foods on your anti-candida diet, you may be able to "starve the yeast" by avoiding refined carbohydrates, sugar, yeast-related products, alcohol, vinegar, and most fermented foods. Some find that they can tolerate one or two pieces of whole fruit per day but fruit juices and dried fruit probably should be avoided. The following table lists foods to be avoided on an anti-candida diet:

FOODS TO AVOID ON ANTI-CANDIDA DIET

Sugar	All types, including honey, maple syrup, barley malt, fructose, date sugar, molasses, corn, cane and beet sugar.
Refined carbohydrates	White flour products, white rice, refined pasta.
Yeast and yeasted products	Yeasted breads, cakes, crackers, muffins, nutritional supplements containing yeast, such as B-complex vitamins, selenium, protein powders, yeast derivatives such as citric acid and MSG.
Alcohol	All types, including cider.
Vinegar and vinegar products	Such as mustard, ketchup, salad dressings, Worcestershire and barbecue sauces, mayonnaise, pickles, sauerkraut, prepared cole slaw.
Fermented foods	Miso, tamari, and soy sauce, tempeh, nuts and nut butter (may contain mold).
Fruit	Including fruit juices and dried fruit.
Dairy	Cow's milk, cheese.
Malted products	Check packaged cereals.
Mold contaminant	Black and herbal teas, dried spices and herbs.
Foods containing steroid or antibiotic residues	Nonorganic meats, chicken, eggs, dairy.

What Are Some Meal Suggestions for a Candida-Free Diet?

SUGGESTED MENU

BREAKFAST

1. Poached organic eggs on wheat-free, yeast-free bread
2. Oat bran cereal with pecans
3. Cooked whole wheat cereal, flaxseed oil, walnuts

LUNCH

1. Lean organic beef patties, 2 toasted rice cakes with homemade hummus, steamed asparagus
2. Broiled chicken breast, 1 cup string beans with almonds, steamed broccoli
3. Tuna fish with lemon and chopped celery, salad with lettuce, tomato, cucumber, carrots, radishes, onions, flaxseed oil and lemon dressing, 2 rice cakes

DINNER

1. Roast organic turkey, small baked potato, steamed cauliflower and broccoli
2. Broiled salmon, baked sweet potato, steamed cabbage, salad with lettuce, tomato, green pepper, and pumpkin seeds with safflower oil and fresh lemon dressing
3. Brown rice with boiled lentils, acorn squash, salad with chopped tomato, onion and basil, steamed green beans

CHAPTER 10

Nutrition Labels: Reading Labels Is Easy

Food labels are filled with so much information that, at times, you may feel you need a dictionary to fully understand the terminology. On the following pages, I will clearly outline the latest terms and definitions that you need to know to help make healthier food selections. Understanding the nutrition facts on your food labels will also help you to make more informed choices.

How Many "Calories from Fat" Are in Your Favorite Food?

Reading labels is essential to maintaining optimal health. To be more knowledgeable about your food selections, it is important to fully understand how to read labels. Labels help identify the number of calories per serving and food constituents. In addition, nutrition labels identify the content of salt, sugar, vitamins, minerals, and fiber. Reading labels will also help you to identify your food allergens.

Ingredients are generally listed in order of the most amount to the least amount. If sugar and a type of fat are the first two ingredients listed on the label, try to use the product sparingly or perhaps not at all. Keep in mind that many of the healthiest foods, such as fresh fruits and vegetables, which are high in fiber, have no cholesterol, and contain only trace amounts of fat, have no food labels at all.

Unfortunately, food labels are far from perfect. The only two vitamins that are required to appear on the label are vitamins A and C. Calcium and iron are the only two minerals that are required on the food label. Obviously, many more key vitamins and minerals are essential in your diet in order to keep you healthy.

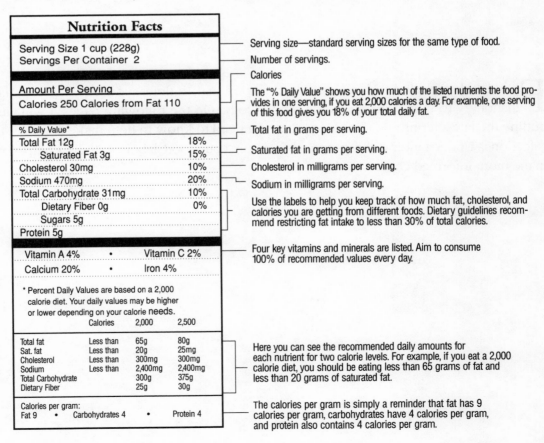

Do You Know the Difference Between Fat-Free and Low-Fat?

The terms and definitions frequently used on food labels and on packages can be very confusing. For example, to understand the difference between *low-fat, light, low-calorie, lean,* and *fat-free* may require in-depth study of food label terminology. Therefore, the following table defines and clarifies the meaning of various food terms.

FOOD LABELS: TERMS AND DEFINITIONS

Cholesterol-free	Less than 2 milligrams of cholesterol and 2 grams or less of saturated fat per serving.
Diet and dietetic	No more than 40 calories per serving or at least a third fewer calories than the regular version of the product.
Enriched and fortified	Added vitamins, minerals, or protein beyond the natural content of those foods.
Extra-lean	Less than 5 grams of fat, 2 grams saturated fat, and 95 milligrams of cholesterol per serving.
Fat-free	Less than 0.5 gram of fat per serving.
Good source of	One serving contains 10–19% of the daily value for that particular nutrient.
High in	One serving contains 20% or more of the daily value for that particular nutrient.
High in polyunsaturates	Products contain vegetable oils other than coconut, palm, or palm kernel oil.
Lean	Less than 10 grams of fat, 4 grams of saturated fat, and 95 milligrams of cholesterol per serving of the meat, poultry, or seafood.
Light or lite	One-third fewer calories or no more than half the fat of the higher-calorie, higher-fat version; or no more than half the sodium of the higher-sodium version.
Low-calorie	40 calories or less per serving.
Low-fat	3 grams or less of saturated fat per serving.
Low-saturated fat	1 gram or less of saturated fat per serving.
Low-sodium	140 milligrams or less of sodium per serving.
No tropical oils	Food must be low in saturated fat because consumers have come to equate tropical oils with high-saturated fat.
Percent fat-free	Food must be low-fat or fat-free and claim must accurately reflect the amount of fat present in 100 grams of the food.
Reduced	The product contains 25% fewer calories or 25% less of a nutrient than the regular product.

Reduced-sodium	The product's salt content has been reduced by at least 25%.
Sodium-free	Less than 5 milligrams of sodium per serving.
Sugar-free	Less than 0.5 gram sugar per serving.
Very low-sodium	35 milligrams or less of sodium per serving.
Juice claims	Beverages which claim to contain juice must list the total percentage of juice.
Implied meanings	A product can no longer imply that it contains a meaningful amount of an ingredient. For example, to make the claim "made with oat bran," the product must contain enough of that ingredient to meet the definition for a "good source" of that ingredient.

CHAPTER 11

Food Storage

No one likes to purchase food only to see it spoil before it is eaten. Storing your food properly can increase shelf life, freshness, and flavor. Moreover, preventing mold buildup and food spoilage can inhibit bacterial contamination of your food. The following pages will identify the length of time various foods can be stored on your shelves, or in your refrigerator or freezer.

DID YOU KNOW THAT:

- Failure to freeze fruits and vegetables immediately after harvest can contribute to losses of vitamins C and E?
- Excessive refrigeration or improper refrigeration can lead to losses of vitamin C and the B-complex vitamins?
- Exposure to light and warm temperatures can cause whole grains, oils, nuts, and seeds to lose valuable quantities of vitamins A, C, and E?
- Storing canned foods at temperatures over 65°F can lead to losses of vitamin C greater than 10 percent; at 80°F, the loss is 25 percent or more?

Can You Store Your Food Forever?

Have you ever wondered how long you can store your pasta, rice, or peanut butter? The following table provides some practical guidelines to keep your food as fresh as possible.

SHELF STORAGE

Food	Maximum Storage Time	Handling Hints
Baking powder	1 year	Keep dry and tightly covered.
Baking soda	1–2 years	Keep dry and tightly covered.
Bread crumbs	6 months	Keep dry and tightly covered.
Cereals: ready-to-eat, unopened	6–12 months	
Cereals: ready-to-eat, opened	2–3 months	Tightly reseal package after each use.
Cereals: to be cooked	6 months	Keep dry and tightly covered.
Cornmeal	1 year	Keep dry and tightly covered.
Cornstarch or arrowroot	18 months	Keep dry and tightly covered.
White flour	2 years	Keep in airtight container.
Grits	1 year	Keep in airtight container.
Honey	1 year	Keep covered.
Nonfat dry milk: unopened	1 year	
Nonfat dry milk: opened	6 months	Keep dry and tightly covered.
Pasta	2+ years	Keep covered.
White rice	2+ years	Keep dry and tightly covered.
Brown rice and rice blends	4–6 months	Keep dry and tightly covered.
Vinegar	2+ years	
Canned foods, unopened	1 year	Keep cool and dry.
Dried fruit, peas and beans	1 year	Store airtight in dark, cool, dry place.
Spices and herbs	6–12 months	Store airtight in dark, cool, dry place.
Fresh onions	6–7 months	Store airtight in dark, cool, dry place.
Peanut butter	6–9 months	Store airtight in dark, cool, dry place.

REFRIGERATOR STORAGE

Food	Maximum Storage Time	Handling Hints
Whole grain flours	4–8 months	Store in moisture-proof, airtight container.
Wheat germ	4–8 months	Store in moisture-proof, airtight container.
Jams and jellies (after opening)	1 year	Keep lids secure.
Oils	3–6 months	Keep well sealed.
Brown sugar	6 months	Store in moisture-proof, airtight container.
Nuts and seeds	6 months	Store in moisture-proof, airtight container.
Butter or margarine	2–4 weeks	Keep covered.
Milk products:		
Cottage cheese	1–2 weeks	Watch for mold or spoilage; keep tightly covered.
Cream cheese	10–14 days	Watch for mold or spoilage; keep tightly covered.
Hard cheese	1–3 weeks	Watch for mold or spoilage; keep tightly covered.
Processed cheese	4–6 weeks	Watch for mold or spoilage; keep tightly covered.
Milk	1 week	Watch for mold or spoilage; keep tightly covered.
Yogurt	3 weeks	Watch for mold or spoilage; keep tightly covered.
Fruit or vegetable juices		
(fresh or reconstituted)	1 week	Keep covered.
Eggs (in shell)	1–2 weeks	Keep covered; will last longer but may lose taste.
Uncooked whole meats:		
(beef, lamb, pork, steaks)	3–5 days	Store in original package.
Ground meat, stew meat, organ meats	1–2 days	Poke a small hole in wrapper to allow for breathing.
Poultry	1–2 days	Store in original package.
Fish	1 day	Store in original package.
Cured and smoked meats:		
Hard sausage	2 weeks	Keep tightly wrapped.
Hot dogs	1 week	Keep tightly wrapped.
Whole ham (fresh)	1 week	Keep tightly wrapped.
Luncheon meats	3–5 days	Keep tightly wrapped.
Canned ham	6–12 months	

PRODUCE STORAGE (STORE UNWASHED AND UNCUT, AS FOLLOWS)

At Room Temperature (Cool, Dry Place)	In Refrigerator "Crisper Drawer"	On Refrigerator Shelf
Avocados[1]	Beets (greens removed)	Apples
Bananas	Broccoli	Apricots
Coconut	Brussels sprouts	Berries[2]
Garlic	Cabbage	Chayote[2]
Guavas[1]	Carrots (leaves removed)	Cherries[2]
Mangos[1]	Cauliflower	Oranges
Onions	Celery	Lemons
Papayas[1]	Corn	Limes
Pineapples[1]	Cucumbers	Grapefruit
Plantains[1]	Eggplant	Coriander (cilantro)[2,3]
Potatoes (white or sweet)	Greens (collard, kale, mustard, escarole, spinach, chicory)	Ginger[2]
Pumpkin, uncut		Grapes[2]
Squash (acorn, butternut, winter)	Jicama	Melons, ripe
Taro	Lettuce	Nectarines[1]
Tomatoes	Mushrooms (in paper bag)	Peaches[1]
Yams	Okra	Plums[1]
Yuca	Peas	Pears[1]
	Peppers	Pumpkin (if cut)
	String beans	Rutabagas
	Turnips	
	Yellow squash	
	Zucchini	

[1] Ripen at room temperature; if ripe, store briefly in refrigerator.
[2] Wrap in plastic.
[3] Wrap wet paper towel around roots.

FREEZER STORAGE

Food	Maximum Storage Time
Prepackaged fruits	1 year
Fruit juice concentrate	1 year
Prepackaged vegetables	8 months
Fruits and vegetables, harvested and fresh frozen	Varies according to type of food and preparation
Bread and rolls	3 months
Cakes (angel, chiffon, chocolate layer) and Danish, pastry, and doughnuts	2–4 months
Fruit pies (unbaked)	8 months
Ice cream and sherbet	1 month
Frozen yogurt	3 days–2 weeks
Uncreamed cottage cheese	1–2 weeks
Hard or semihard cheese	6–12 months
Soft cheese	4 months
Heavy cream	3–6 months
Milk	1 month
Butter	5–6 months
Prepackaged frozen meat	3 months
Fresh frozen meat:	
Beef steaks, roast, lamb	9–12 months
Ground beef and veal	4–6 months
Pork	6–9 months
Pork sausage	1–3 months
Beef or lamb liver	3–4 months
Pork liver	1–2 months
Bacon slab and whole ham	1–3 months
Prepackaged frozen poultry:	
Whole	12 months
Cut up	9 months
Livers	3 months
Whole duck or goose	6 months
Turkey, whole	12 months
Turkey, cut up	6 months
Precooked frozen poultry dinners or pies	6 months
Fried chicken	4 months

Food	Maximum Storage Time
Poultry (fresh):	
Chicken, duck, game birds	6–7 months
Giblets	2–3 months
Turkey	4–5 months
Geese	3–4 months
Frozen packaged fish:	
Fillets (cod, flounder, haddock, halibut)	6 months
Fillets (mullet, ocean perch, sea trout, striped bass)	3 months
Whole ocean perch and salmon steaks	2 months
Sea trout and striped bass	3 months
Fresh-caught and frozen fish	4–6 months
Shellfish:	
Clams, shucked	3 months
Dungeness crab	3 months
King crab	10 months
Oysters, shucked	4 months
Shrimp	1 year
Frozen fish dinners, fish sticks	3 months

Part II

ALLERGIES

CHAPTER 12

Food Allergies from A to Z

A food allergy is often defined as an immediate adverse reaction to a food caused by the release of a specific immunoglobulin or antibody known as "IgE." Classic food allergy reactions are immediate and may manifest with hives, wheezing, or other symptoms.

Food intolerances or sensitivities are abnormal reactions to commonly ingested substances. They may also result from repeated and cumulative exposures to a commonly eaten food, frequently combined with a weakened immune response.

Could Your Colitis Be Due to Food Allergies?

Whereas the term "food allergy" refers to the release of IgE antibodies, the term "food intolerance" refers to adverse reactions to foods that include mechanisms other than the production of IgE antibodies. Both food allergies and food intolerances may produce the same or similar symptoms. These symptoms can affect any part of your body. It may be necessary to avoid ingesting the foods that are causing your adverse reactions.

What Are the Two Main Types of Food Reactions?

Immediate
- Potentially life-threatening (5% of food reactions).
- Involves IgE cells of the immune system.
- Involves release of histamine.
- These reactions are relatively rare.

Delayed
- Reactions can occur anywhere from a few hours to a few days later.
- May be difficult to identify due to delay in symptoms.
- These reactions to foods are the most common.

Food allergies or sensitivities can affect vitually any part of your body—from your head to your toes. This does not mean that the symptoms listed below are always caused by reactions to foods; however, these symptoms have at times been associated with food reactions. In fact, I would estimate that nearly 60 percent of the chronic, undiagnosed problems that my patients experience have food allergies that may be causing, contributing to, or exacerbating their symptoms.

HOW FOOD REACTIONS CAN AFFECT YOUR BODY

Body Part	Reactions
Eyes Ears Nose Throat	Dark circles or swelling and wrinkles under eyes, nasal congestion, excessive mucus, postnasal drip, watery eyes, blurred vision, tinnitus, earaches, hearing loss, repeated throat or ear infections, ear itching, sore throats, hoarseness, chronic cough, canker sores, recurrent sinusitis.
Head	Headaches, faintness, dizziness, excessive drowsiness after eating, insomnia.
Heart and lungs	Palpitations, arrhythmias, rapid heart rate, asthma, chest congestion.
Gastrointestinal	Mucus in stools, undigested food, nausea, vomiting, diarrhea, constipation, bloating, belching, colitis, flatulence, abdominal pains or cramps, irritable bowel syndrome, colic in infants, extreme thirst, Crohn's disease and ulcerative colitis, rectal itching.
Genitourinary	Urinary frequency or urgency, vaginal discharge or itching, PMS, chronic cystitis, bed wetting.
Musculoskeletal	Swelling, aches and pains of joints and/or muscles.
Psychological symptoms	Anxiety, panic attacks, depression, crying spells, aggressiveness, irritability, confusion, hyperactivity, restlessness, learning disabilities, slurred speech, concentration difficulty.
Skin	Hives, rashes, eczema, pallor, dry skin, dandruff, brittle nails and hair.
Other symptoms	Chronic fatigue, "growing pains" in children, food cravings, obesity, daily weight fluctuation, certain types of autism.

Which Foods Most Commonly Cause Food Allergies?

In my clinical experience, eggs, yeast, wheat, milk, corn, and soy make up the six most common offending foods that contribute to food allergies. If you are allergic or sensitive to foods, abstain from eating them in all forms until you have developed a tolerance to them. By avoiding the offending food, you can place your immune system at rest, thus allowing it to repair itself. Abstaining from the food for two to four months may be all you need to gain tolerance.

Initially, you may experience cravings or withdrawal symptoms such as anxiety, tension, light-headedness, headaches, or fatigue after you have eliminated an offending food but these symptoms should resolve after the first week. If, however, you have a strong IgE-mediated food allergy reaction including breathing difficulties, hives, or shortness of breath, you should avoid this food at all costs.

The following table lists six of the most common foods contributing to food allergies and sensitivities and where these foods may be hidden. As you can imagine, reading labels is extremely important if you are troubled by food allergies. Did you realize that both spaghetti and pretzels may contain eggs? Or that most commercial soups, breads, and cereals contain soy? If you suffer from allergies to any of the six foods listed, be aware that they can be hidden in many other foods.

MOST COMMON SOURCES OF FOOD ALLERGIES

Egg	Yeast	Wheat		Milk	Corn		Soybean
Baking powders	Barbecue sauce	Alcoholic	Cocoa	Au gratin	Ales	Catsup	Baby foods
Bavarian cream	Barley cereal	beverages	Cookies	foods	Aspirin	Chewing gum	Biscuits
Breaded foods	Beer	Baby foods	Cooked meat	Bavarian	Bacon	Coffee	Breads
Breads	Brandy	Barley malt	dishes	cream	Baking	Cough syrups	Butter
Cake flours	Breads	Batter (for fried	Chocolate	Biscuits	powder	Corn chips	substitutes
Cakes	Buns	foods)	candy	Breads	Beers	Cream pies	Cakes
French toast	Buttermilk	Beer, gin,	Cold cuts	Butter	Biscuits	Cured hams	Caramel
Fritters	Cakes	whiskey	Corn bread	Buttermilk	Bleached	Dates	Cereals
Frostings	Canned mince	Biscuits	Crackers	Cakes	flour	(confections)	Cheese
Frying batters	meat	Bisquick	Cream of	Cookies	Bourbon	Distilled vine-	Coffee
Glazed rolls	Cereals	Bologna	wheat	Candy	Breads	gar	substitutes
Griddle cakes	Cheeses	Bouillon cubes	Croutons	Cheese	Pastries	Doughnuts	Crackers
Hamburger mix	Chili peppers	Bran	Doughnuts	Chocolate	Cakes	Frostings	Hard candy
Hollandaise sauce	Citrus fruit	Breads	Dumplings	Chowders	Cereals	Frozen fruits	Ice cream
Ice cream	juices	Bread crumbs	Farina	Cocoa drinks	Cookies	Frozen	Lecithin
Icings	Condiments	Breaded	Flour	Creamed	Cheeses	vegetables	Lunch meats
Macaroni	Cookies	products	Gluten	foods	Candy	Fruits (canned	Margarine
Macaroons	Cottage cheese	Bread stuffing	Graham	Creamed	Chop suey	and frozen)	substitutes
Marshmallows	Crackers	Bulgur	products	sauces	Chili	Fat frying	Milk substitutes
Mayonnaise	Enriched flours	Cakes	Granola	Curds	Carbonated	batters	Miso
Meat loaf	Fruit juices	Cereals	Gravies	Custards	beverages	Gelatins	Nut candies

MOST COMMON SOURCES OF FOOD ALLERGIES (cont.)

Egg	Yeast	Wheat		Milk	Corn		Soybean
Meringues	Gin	Griddle cakes	Pastries	Doughnuts	Grape juice	Salad dressing	Oils
Noodles	Horseradish	Hamburger	Pies	Flour mixes	Glucose products	Sandwich	Oriental sauces
Pancake	Ketchup	mix	Pita	Fritters	Graham crackers	spreads	Pastries
flour	Malted milk	Hot dogs	pockets	Gravies	Gravies	Sausage	Pork link
Pancakes	products	Ice cream	Pizza	Hamburger mix	Grits	Sherbet	sausages
Pretzels	Mayonnaise	Liverwurst	Pretzels	Hash	Ham (cured)	Soups (creamed)	Salad dressings
Puddings	Mince pie	Macaroni	Puddings	Ice cream	Ice cream	Soy bean milk	Soups
Salad dress-	Mushrooms	Malt products	Sausages	Margarine	Sherbets	Starch	Soy flour
ings	Olives	Matzoh	Soups	Mashed potatoes	Instant teas	Toothpaste	Soy noodles
Sauces	Pastries	Mayonnaise	Soy sauce	Omelets	Jellies	Tortillas	Soy macaroni
Sausages	Pickles	Muffins	Spaghetti	Ovaltine	Margarine	Vegetables	Soy sauces
Sherbets	Pretzels	Noodles	Tortillas	Ovamalt	Pancake mix	(canned,	Soy sprouts
Soufflés	Rum	Pancake mix	Waffles	Pancakes	Peanut butter	frozen,	Tempura
Soups	Salad dress-	Pasta	Yeast	Pie crusts	Pie crusts	creamed)	Tofu
Spaghetti	ing			Rarebits	Popcorn	Vanilla	Worcestershire
Tartar sauce	Sauerkraut			Salad dressing	Powdered sugars	Vitamins	sauce
Waffles/mix	Soy sauce			Sausages	Preserves	Whiskey	
Wine	Tomato sauce			(cooked)	Puddings and		
	Truffles			Scalloped	custard		
	Vinegar			potatoes			
	Vodka			Sherbets			
	Vitamins			Soda crackers			
	Whiskey			Soufflés			
	Wine			Soups (creamed)			
	Yogurt			Spumoni			
				Waffles			
				Whey			
				Yogurt			

Sources: Adapted from Jacqueline Krohn, *The Whole Way to Allergy Relief and Prevention*, and Immuno Laboratories, Inc.

You're Not Alone in Your Allergy to Milk!

As I have mentioned, the foods most commonly associated with causing allergies include corn, eggs, milk, soy, wheat, yeast, and sugar. Some foods such as carrots or lamb are rarely associated with food allergies. The following table lists a variety of foods, from those most likely to those least likely to cause allergic reactions, in order of frequency.

FREQUENCY OF COMMON FOOD ALLERGIES

Most Common	Often	Sometimes	Seldom
Corn	Alcohol	Alfalfa	Apricots
Eggs	Apples	Amaranth	Beets
Milk	Bacon	Bananas	Carrots
Soy	Beans, dried	Barley (malt)	Cranberries
Sugar	Beef	Celery	Grapes
Wheat	Berries	Cherry	Honey
Yeast	Buckwheat	Chicken	Lamb
	Cheese	Chilis	Peaches
	Chocolate	Cloves	Rabbit
	Cinnamon	Cottonseed	Salmon
	Coconut	Garlic	Salt
	Coffee	Lobster	Squash
	Fish	Melon	Sweet potato
	Lettuce	Mushrooms	Tapioca
	Mustard	Oats	Taro root
	Nuts	Oysters	Tea
	Onions	Pears	Vanilla
	Oranges (citrus)	Peppers	
	Peanuts	Pineapples	
	Peas	Plums	
	Pork	Prunes	
	Potatoes	Quince	
	Raisins	Rice	
	Rye	Sesame seeds	
	Shrimp	Spices	
	Tomatoes	Spinach	
		Strawberries	
		Sunflowers	
		Turkey	
		Vinegar	

Does Your Child Have Food Allergies?

Food allergy or food sensitivity in children is not uncommon. Many infants and young children appear to outgrow allergies to food and formula when, in fact, the allergy is simply in a period of transition. Their allergies may manifest at a later time in life, in a different part of the body. For example, an infant with allergies to formula may develop asthma at age six and then headaches at age ten.

The prevention of food allergies actually begins upon conception and continues with the development of the fetus. During pregnancy, it is essential for the mother-to-be to be conscientious about food selections in order to minimize her child's susceptibility to food allergy. For example, I frequently advise pregnant women who have a history of food allergies to rotate their own food intake during pregnancy if possible. This reduces the likelihood of the unborn baby developing food allergies after birth. A baby's diet, like the adult diet, should also be varied in order to avoid food allergies. Mothers who breastfeed should also be aware that by repetitively eating the same foods, they may make their infants more susceptible to food allergies. For this reason, breastfeeding mothers should also try to rotate their food intake.

Incidentally, breastfeeding is a wonderful way of boosting your child's immune system and protecting him or her from future illnesses. Breast milk is rich in immunoglobulin and other immune factors, which can help strengthen your child's immune response. Breast-feeding is also a way for the new mom to bond with her baby and to provide top-quality nutrition. Breastfeeding may also help the nursing mother lose her pregnancy weight faster and to protect her from bone loss and breast cancer. If possible, I would suggest trying to nurse for at least six months and more optimally strive to breastfeed for a full year. You should discuss these issues with your pediatrician should you have concerns or questions. I have found that a lactation specialist or nurse-midwife is generally well educated and quite informative in instructing you on the proper nursing techniques or dealing with problems should they arise.

Symptoms of food allergy vary throughout the stages of development from infancy to adolescence. Typically, within an hour after eating the problem food, the child can develop red earlobes and cheeks, dark circles under the eyes, an inability to sit still, a "spaced-out" look, a sudden personality change, or other health complaints. Following are typical age-related symptoms of food allergy. If your child exhibits any of these symptoms, food allergies may be the culprit.

SYMPTOMS OF FOOD ALLERGIES IN CHILDREN

Infancy

Prolonged screaming and crying, excessive spitting up, constant desire to be fed, head banging, irritability, reluctance to be held, nonstop drooling, eczema, colic, diarrhea, constipation, poor sleep patterns, crib rocking, infrequent smiling, recurrent ear infections, congestion, sweating, walking before ten months.

Toddlers

Temper tantrums, leg cramps, behavior problems, fatigue, asthma, headaches, intestinal complaints, earaches, hyperactivity, stuffy nose, throat clearing, chronic cough, crawling in dark corners, and refusal to be touched.

Children

Hayfever, clucking throat sounds, diarrhea or constipation, inconsistent school performance, recurrent infections, asthma, headaches, leg cramps, sudden mood and behavior changes, inability to write or draw, hives, eczema, and bedwetting after age 5.

Adolescents

Fatigue, depression, irritability, poor memory, diarrhea, constipation or gas, aggression, moodiness, easy crying, chronic asthma, hayfever, sinusitis, bloating, chronic bowel disease, bad breath, and hives.

Do You Have Hidden Food Intolerances?

Food intolerances do not involve the classic IgE antibody production or release associated with food allergies. They are commonly triggered by other immunologic reactions or may even be caused by reactions to other substances.

For example, an individual may have an adverse reaction to shellfish but test negative with classic IgE or traditional skin allergy testing. Other mechanisms may account for his adverse reaction to ingesting shellfish. For example, mercury sensitivity may be the real culprit responsible for the adverse reaction to shellfish.

Another example would be a naturally occurring histamine found in foods such as cheese, sauerkraut, and wine, which can be responsible for adverse reactions to these foods. Additives or food contaminants may also contribute to food intolerances.

In the following tables, you will find examples of substances that may cause adverse reactions or intolerances to foods. In these cases, traditional skin testing or an allergy blood test measuring only IgE antibodies would typically come out negative and you may be told that you are not allergic to the food. However, owing to other mechanisms that cause food reactions, you may still be intolerant to that particular food.

NATURALLY OCCURRING FOOD CHEMICALS

Foods containing certain naturally occurring chemicals may cause problems for susceptible individuals.

Food	Chemical Culprit
Citrus fruits	Salicylates, octopamine
Potatoes	Solanidines
Rhubarb	Oxalic acid
Peas and beans	Lecitins
Fruit kernels	Cyanide
Millet and cabbage	Gointrogens
Mushrooms	Alkaloids

FOOD ADDITIVES

Food additives in various products have been shown to cause adverse reactions.

Food	Chemical
Soft drinks, sweets, orange juice, yellow artificially colored foods	Tartrazine
Processed foods	Benzoic acid
Soy sauce, meat extract, wine, Chinese foods, yeast extracts	Glutamate
Processed meats, pork, cheese, hot dogs, pickles	Nitrates
Vegetables, wine	Metabisulfite
Wine, beer, spirits	Alcohol
Soft drinks, jams, jellies, cakes, biscuits, pastry	Azo dyes
Oils, food cooked in oil, margarine	Preservatives BHA and BHT
Yeast extracts	Brewer's yeast

Food Toxins

Some foods may have naturally occurring food toxins, while others become toxic through storage and processing.

Food	Toxin
Grains	Bacteria and fungus
Peanuts	Mycotoxins and aflatoxins
Fermented foods	Mold toxins
Fish	Soxitoxin
Shellfish	Scromboid poisoning, cigualera poisoning, mercury

Naturally Occurring Amines

Foods can contain naturally occurring chemical compounds known as amines, which can be responsible for adverse reactions to foods.

Food	Amine
Coffee, tea	Caffeine
Tuna, cheese, pork, sauerkraut, wine	Histamine
Cheese, red wine, pickled herring, liver	Tyramine
Bananas	Serotonin
Chocolate, cola, cocoa	Theobromine

Infectious Food Organisms

Foods can be contaminated with infectious agents such as bacteria, parasites, and viruses.

Organism	Disease
Bacteria	Botulism
	Salmonellosis
	Staphylococcal
	Intoxication
Parasites	Amoeba
	Giardiasis
	Trichinosis
Viruses	Hepatitis

Food Contaminants (Accidental)

Many foods are contaminated with substances that may cause problems for some individuals.

Food	Accidental Contaminant
Mercury in oysters, can linings	Heavy metals
Fruits, vegetables, grains	Pesticides
Milk	Antibiotics (penicillin, tetracycline, bacitracin), steroids
Plastic wrappings	Formaldehyde, benzoates, and sodium bisulphate

Is Your Glass of Wine Contributing to Your Allergies?

Many allergens are found in the foods from which alcohol is made: sugar, yeast, grain, and corn being the most common. Allergic reactions can intensify a genetic predisposition to an addiction, or the allergen itself may be the cause of the addiction. Therefore, it is believed that food allergy may play a significant role in alcohol addiction. The following table gives examples of common allergens found in alcoholic beverages.

ALLERGENS FOUND IN ALCOHOLIC BEVERAGES

Key
- ● = commonly used
- + = less frequently used or used in smaller quantities

	CORN (A)	BARLEY MALT	RYE (B)	WHEAT (C)	OATS	RICE	POTATO	GRAPES	PLUM	CITRUS	APPLE	PEAR	PEACH	CHERRY	HOPS	CACTUS	BEET SUGAR	CANE SUGAR	YEAST
Wines																			
Grape	●							●									●	●	●
Champagne								●									●	●	●
Vermouth	+	+	+	+	+			●									●	●	●
Sherry	●							●									●	●	●
Cider	●										●						●	●	●
Malt Beverages																			
Beer	●	●	+	+	+	●									●				●
Ale	●	●	+	+	+	●									●				●
Flavored beer	●	●	+	+	+	●		●		●					●				●
Whiskey																			
Straight (corn, bourbon, malt, rye)	●	●	●	●	●	●													●
Blended(d) (corn, bourbon, malt, rye)	●	●	●	●	●	●													●
Canadian, blended	●	●	●	●					●	●	●						+	●	
Scotch whiskey, unblended	+	●															+	+	
Scotch whiskey, blended(d)	●	●															+	+	
Irish whiskey, unblended		●	●	●	●													+	●
Irish whiskey, blended(d)		●	●	●	●	●			●	●	●						+	+	●
Gin																			
Grain spirits	●	●	●	+	+	+				●						●	+	+	●
Cane spirits(e)																		●	●
Flavored	●	●	●	●	●	●	●	●	●	●	●	●	●	●	●	●	+	+	●

Key

- ● = commonly used
- + = less frequently used or used in smaller quantities

	CORN (A)	BARLEY MALT	RYE (B)	WHEAT (C)	OATS	RICE	POTATO	GRAPES	PLUM	CITRUS	APPLE	PEAR	PEACH	CHERRY	HOPS	CACTUS	BEET SUGAR	CANE SUGAR	YEAST
Vodka																			
Domestic	●	●	●	●	●			●											●
Imported																			
Flavored	●	●	●	●	●	●	●	●	●	●	●	●	●	●	●	●			●
Rum																			
Domestic (includes Puerto Rican rum)								●										●	●
Jamaican																		●	●
Tequila																●		●	●
Liqueurs	●	●	+	+	+	+	+	●	●	●	●	●	●	●	●	●		●	●
Brandy																			
Grape	+							●									+	+	●
Cognac								+									+	+	●
Applejack	+										●						+	+	●
Blackberry	+																+	+	●

Notes:

a. Although the practice of adding corn sugar to wine for fermentation is common, wines produced in California are guaranteed free of added sugars if they carry the "Made in California" label.

b. Many people who are sensitive to wheat are either sensitive to rye or readily become so if rye is employed as a wheat substitute.

c. If you are sensitive to wheat, the chances are extremely high that you will also show a sensitivity to malt (sprouted dried barley).

d. Blended whiskeys, the less expensive ones at least, are more apt to contain potato spirits.

e. Cane spirits and gin also contain hops, mint, and/or herbs.

Source: Theron G. Randolph, M.D.

CHAPTER 13

Inhalant Allergies: Nothing to Sneeze at

Inhalants are airborne substances small enough to be inhaled through the nose, then into the lungs. They are found in your everyday environment, your home, your workplace, and your school. After absorption by the lining of the respiratory tract, these allergens can be carried to other body organs and cause symptoms at other distant sites.

It is well known that pollens derived from grasses, trees, and weeds, as well as dust, molds, feathers, and animal hair and dander, can cause respiratory allergy or "hay fever" in susceptible individuals. Nasal congestion, sneezing, watery eyes, coughing, and asthma can result from inhaling these allergens.

Symptoms of Inhalant Allergies

- Hoarseness
- Sneezing
- Increased mucus production
- Scratchy throat
- Runny nose

- Hay fever
- Itchy, watery eyes
- Hives
- Facial tenderness
- Eczema
- Insomnia

- Fatigue
- Swollen glands
- Asthma
- Panic attacks
- Diarrhea
- Skipped heartbeats

Under What Conditions Might Your Inhalant Allergies Get Better or Worse?

Pollens

Symptoms May Be Better:

- On rainy days
- Indoors, with air conditioning
- After first light frost

Symptoms May Be Worse:

- On clear, windy days
- When going from air conditioning to open air
- During peak pollen seasons

Dust

Symptoms May Be Better:

- Outdoors

Symptoms May Be Worse

- Indoors
- While dusting and cleaning
- When the furnace is turned on in cold weather
- Minutes after going to bed
- When the house is sealed because air conditioning or heat is on

Molds

Symptoms May Be Better:

- Inside when air conditioning or heat is on
- When snow is on the ground

Symptoms May Be Worse:

- In cool evening air
- In damp places
- When cutting grass or raking leaves
- From September to frost

Treatment for inhalant allergies may include allergy testing, allergy desensitization, environmental control, antihistamines, decongestants, other medications, natural supplements, herbal remedies, and avoidance of the inhalant whenever possible.

Pollens

Over 15 million individuals suffer from allergic reactions to pollens. The release of pollen can vary depending on your geographic location, the time of year, the time of day, the weather conditions, and changes in the weather. Weeds are the most important cause of hay fever and probably produce the greatest amounts of pollen. Ragweed is the most well known of the weed group and is the most potent in producing allergy symptoms. Grasses are all morphologically similar to each other, and also release significant amounts of pollen. Pollens are difficult to avoid in warm weather, and it may be advisable to stay in an air-conditioned room. HEPA (high efficiency particulate accumulator) air purifiers can also reduce the amount of pollens inside your home, car, or office.

When Do Trees, Grasses, and Weeds Pollinate in Your Region?

The time of year in which trees, grasses, and weeds pollinate in your part of the country can vary greatly. As you can see from the table below, there is a great differential between pollen seasons whether you live in the Northeastern part of the United States compared to, for example, the Western states such as California and Nevada. Use the general guidelines in the following table to become more familiar with the various pollen seasons.

REGION	POLLINATION MONTHS		
	Trees	Grass	Weeds
Northeast, Mid-Atlantic (Maine, New Hampshire, Vermont, Rhode Island, New York, Massachusetts, Connecticut, New Jersey, Delaware, West Virginia, Maryland, and Pennsylvania)	February–July	February–September	April–October
Southeast (Virginia, North Carolina, South Carolina, Georgia, Florida, Alabama, Louisiana, Mississippi, Arkansas, Tennessee, and Kentucky)	December–October	January–October	April–October
North Central (Minnesota, Wisconsin, Iowa, Michigan, Missouri, Illinois, Indiana, and Ohio)	December–July	February–September	April–October
Central (North Dakota, South Dakota, and Nebraska)	February–July	February–October	April–October
South Central (Kansas, Oklahoma, and Texas)	January–October	January–October	March–October
Southwest (Arizona, New Mexico, Utah, and Colorado)	January–October	January–October	March–October
Central Northwest (Idaho, Montana, and Wyoming)	February–July	March–September	April–September

REGION	POLLINATION MONTHS		
	Trees	Grass	Weeds
Northwest (Washington and Oregon)	February–September	February–August	March–November
Western (California and Nevada)	January–October	January–October	March–November
Alaska	March–July	April–August	May–September
Hawaii	Varies	Varies	Varies

Molds

Are You Sensitive to Mold in Your Bathroom or Kitchen?

Molds are present in your indoor and outdoor environments, and can also be a cause of common allergic symptoms. Molds are usually associated with nasal congestion, sneezing, itchy eyes, and excessive mucus. They flourish in damp weather conditions and are present indoors and outdoors during the entire year. Allergenic reactions to mold can also prompt depression, insomnia, and skin disorders including psoriasis, eczema, or skin yeast in many patients.

What Are the Characteristics of Molds?

- Widespread on foods and plants
- Found in soil and air
- Spores spread by wind, insects, and humans
- Midsummer through fall are peak months to multiply
- Grow best at 70°–90°F
- Leave musty smell indoors

COMMON MOLDS AND THEIR SOURCES

Alternaria	Grows on plants, plant materials, fruits, vegetables, and cereal grains.
Aspergillus	Common soil fungus on damp hay, grains, fruits, and sausage. Common on wet surfaces in bathrooms and in drip pans of refrigerators and other appliances. Grows on stored food products under damp conditions.
Botrytis	Found on garden flowers during wet weather.
Cephalosporium	Commonly found in soil and as a component of dust in textile factories.
Epicoccum	Found on decaying vegetative materials, plant leaves, and uncooked fruit.
Fomes	Found on rotting wood.
Fusarium	Found on green plants such as peas, beans, tomatoes, corn, sweet potatoes, rice, and cotton.
Geotrichum	Commonly found in soil and milk.
Helminthosporium	Found on cereal grains such as corn, wheat, oats, and rye.
Hormodendrum	Found on decomposing plants, leather, rubber, cloth, paper, and wood products. Spores are released in great numbers after rain and damp weather. Found around barns and barnyards where it grows on animal waste.
Penicillin	Normally a soil inhabitant but grows on fruits, breads, cheese, and other foods. Mutant strains are used to produce the antibiotic penicillin.
Phoma	Grows on paper products such as books and magazines. Also grows on certain plants.
Pullularia	Found in soil but grows on decaying vegetation, plants, and chalking compounds.
Rhizopus	Grows on bread, cured meats, root vegetables, and indoors on stored sugary food products including bakery goods, fruit, and sweet potatoes.
Rhodotorula	Common soil inhabitant.
Sporobolomyces	Found on wood decay on forest trees.
Stemphylium	Grows on damp paper, canvas, and cotton fabric, as well as decaying plant material.
Trichoderma	Found mainly on decaying wood. Also grows on damp cotton and wool. May be found in damp basements.

Source: William Rea, M.D.

How Can You Control Indoor Mold Naturally?

It is essential to reduce your exposure to mold. Consider the following as an adjunct to your treatment.

NATURAL METHODS TO CONTROL MOLD

- Sprinkle borax powder in mold-prone areas, like the bottom of the garbage can. Also add ½ cup to your wash load in addition to your laundry detergent.
- Discourage musty odors by adding vinegar to your wash load.
- Zephiran concentrate acts as a fungicide and a germicide. Use 1 ounce to 1 gallon of water.
- Activated charcoal can be used to absorb odors.
- Turn on lights to discourage mold growth. Use night lights, even in the bathroom.
- Circulate the air using small electric fans or ceiling fans to discourage mold growth.
- Get rid of dampness using fans or lights under the house to discourage mold. Have the ground under the house lined with plastic.
- Keep clothes clean by never hanging them in the closet after they have been worn. Mold grows on them. Also, keep closets, dresser drawers, bathrooms, and refrigerator as clean and dry as possible.
- Dry shower curtain and tub area with a small fan to reduce mold growth. Leave a light on in the shower to discourage mold.
- Refrigerator drip tray and rubber door gasket should be cleaned.
- Wet towels and washcloths should be taken immediately to laundry area or hung outside to dry if you have to postpone laundering.
- Change pet litter daily to reduce mold growth. Better yet, keep your cat out of the house altogether.
- Throw out all damp piles of odds and ends you have been hoarding (newspapers, books, magazines, old carpets, cast-off furniture, old worn pillows, etc.).
- Use only light, washable throw rugs instead of heavy carpeting. Carpet is a lush haven for mold growth.
- Avoid using wallpaper, especially in the bathroom to minimize mold.
- Replace old mattresses, a source of mold. Regularly air newer mattresses to discourage musty odors.
- Check your rainspout, and extend the downspout to carry rainwater farther away from house.
- Put plants outside because the soil contains mold.

TIPS

If you are mold-sensitive, it is advisable to avoid fermented foods:
- Buttermilk, cheeses, mushrooms, pickles, processed spices, sauerkraut, sour cream, tofu, and vinegar.
- Fermented beverages: beer, cider, wine.

Part III

OUR CHEMICAL ENVIRONMENT

CHAPTER 14

Chemical Exposures

*Up to 75 million American workers are at risk of
becoming ill because of the buildings they work in.*
—The Environmental Protection Agency (EPA)

Our indoor and outdoor environments have become a major source of chemical pollution. Our food and water supply have also become contaminated with chemicals. As a result of this constant exposure, a significant percentage of our population is becoming sensitized to chemicals, thereby triggering a host of clinical complaints. Chemical sensitivities are becoming more prevalent with each passing decade owing to the increase of chemical exposures.

Most people seem to tolerate low levels of chemical exposure without difficulty. However, there is a small but growing segment of the population who, unfortunately, is unable to cope with exposure to even minute quantities of chemical agents. Once you have become sensitized to chemicals, you may begin to react adversely to other irritants that were previously thought to be harmless. You may also develop symptoms from exposures to chemicals at levels that are usually tolerated by the majority of individuals. Your ability to adapt to and tolerate these chemicals decreases with frequent exposures, and your symptoms may eventually become more chronic and persistent.

Severe reactions may result from a massive exposure to particular chemicals, such as those found in pesticides or herbicides, those found in anesthesia, and those found in a chemical spill. Adverse reactions may also result from repeated, low-level exposures to common chemicals such as exhaust fumes, air pollution, outgassing from new building materials, scented soaps and detergents, disinfectants, cleaning agents, cigarette smoke, paints, insecticides, pesticides, and perfumes. When these exposures are coupled with a weakened immune system, a predisposition to certain genetic factors, or inadequate detoxification mechanisms, it can result in a chronic medical condition known as multiple chemical sensitivity (MCS). According to a National Academy of Sciences workshop, it has been estimated that 15 percent of our population has chemical sensitivities.

What Are the Symptoms of Chemical Sensitivities?

Some individuals experiencing poor health may not be aware that chemical sensitivities are playing a role in their illness. Because toxicity is often cumulative, symptoms can be delayed, difficult to identify, and therefore erroneously attributed to other causes. Just like food allergy symptoms, symptoms of chemical sensitivities can also affect virtually every organ system in the body. The following table will identify some of the more common symptoms associated with chemical exposures.

SYMPTOMS OF CHEMICAL SENSITIVITIES

Cerebral Symptoms
- Anger
- Depression
- Disorientation
- Concentration problems
- Apathy
- Emotional instability
- Headache
- Light-headedness
- Mental fatigue

Ear, Nose, and Throat Symptoms
- Ringing in the ears
- Coughing
- Itching in the ears
- Rhinitis
- Nasal obstruction
- Stuffy nose

Eye Symptoms
- Vision disturbances
- Watery eyes
- Light sensitivity
- Itching
- Swollen or red eyelids

Gastrointestinal and Urinary Symptoms
- Diarrhea
- Constipation
- Frequent urination
- Vomiting
- Nausea
- Gas
- Dry mouth
- Abdominal pain
- Heartburn
- Gallbladder symptoms

Musculoskeletal Symptoms
- Fatigue
- Muscle cramps
- Weakness
- Joint pain or stiffness
- Lack of coordination

Respiratory Symptoms
- Coughing
- Asthma

Are You Being Bombarded by Chemical Pollutants?

Although new governmental regulations have tried to improve air quality, you may be surprised to learn that indoor air often poses a more serious health hazard than outdoor air to susceptible individuals. If you notice adverse reactions when exposed to the following pollutants, you may want to ask your doctor about a chemical pollution defense program which includes an antioxidant protocol, an immune enhancement program, a desensitization treatment protocol, and/or a chemical avoidance plan.

OUTDOOR CHEMICAL POLLUTANTS

Drinking water

Fuel combustion and smelters

Industrial emissions

Insecticide and pesticide sprays

Oil refineries and storage tanks

Oil-derived solvents

Road paving and resurfacing

Photochemical reactions

Smog

Smoke from fireplaces and wood stoves

Tarring roofs

Traffic exhaust

Trees, grass, weeds, and flowers

Vaporization of unburned fuels

INDOOR CHEMICAL STRESSORS

- FUEL-BASED PRODUCTS—give off toxic end products of combustion and can leak through walls and floors.
- NATURAL GAS—can leak from gas ranges, refrigerators, dryers, and water heaters.
- OIL FUMES—can escape from garages, furnaces, appliances, and oil-soaked filters from air conditioners.
- FORCED HOT AIR SYSTEMS—are conducive to the growth of molds and to the passage of dust.

The home, school, and workplace can all be a source of chemical hazards that can adversely affect your health. Construction materials such as fiberboard, paneling, plywood, and fiberglass, as well as carpets and building foam insulation, all contain large amounts of formaldehyde. Chemicals from fresh paint, insecticides, disinfectants, flooring waxes as well as outgassing from computers, copy machines, carbon paper, and other office supplies, can become trapped in "energy-efficient" buildings with nonoperational windows, contributing to poor indoor air quality and what is referred to as "sick-building syndrome." Proper ventilation and air filtration are perhaps the most important factors to eliminate "sick-building syndrome" and to reduce your total load of chemical exposures.

> *Indoor air pollution is one of the greatest health threats of all environmental problems. It ranks as the fourth highest cancer risk and poses the third greatest risk to human health.*
>
> —The Environmental Protection Agency (EPA)

What Are the Most Prevalent Indoor Chemical Stressors?

If your symptoms seem to be triggered or exacerbated by your home or work environment, a detailed history and a careful evaluation of your surroundings are essential. The following table may help you identify the chemical irritants in your home or office. Another new concern is that schools are now also increasingly becoming sources of chemical exposures. All too often, we attribute common symptoms such as mental fatigue, dizziness, headaches, nasal congestion, or irritated eyes to cold symptoms or viruses when, in fact, these symptoms might be caused by a variety of indoor air pollutants. If you experience an increase in symptoms when you are exposed to any of the following indoor chemical stressors, you may have chemical sensitivities.

INDOOR CHEMICAL IRRITANTS

Aerosols
Air deodorizers
Aluminum pots and pans
Ammonia
Animal dander
Asbestos (fire-retardant materials, insulation)

Bleaches

Car exhaust fumes
Cedar-lined closets
Charcoal
Chlorinated or fluoridated water
Cleaning products
Cosmetics

Dust, dust mites
Deodorants, antiperspirants
Detergents
Disinfectants
Dyes

Electric blankets

Felt-tip pens
Flameproof mattresses
Floor cleaners and waxes
Food additives
Formaldehyde
Fungicide-treated wallpaper
Furniture polish

Gas stoves and gas appliances

Hair sprays
Heat-sealed soft plastic packages

Insecticides

Kerosene

Lacquer
Lubricants
Medications
Mineral oil
Mothballs and moth crystals
Mothproofed shelf paper
Mouthwash
Mold

Nail polish
Newsprint

Oven cleaners

Paint fumes
Paraffin
Perfumes, aftershaves
Permanent-press clothing
Pesticides
Pine-scented cleaners
Plastic food containers and plastic wraps
Plastics (mattress covers, tablecloths, shower curtains, draperies, food wrappers, shelf paper)

Radon
Refrigerant gas
Rubber-backed carpets
Rubbing alcohol

Scented soap
Shampoo
Solvents
Smoke
Sponge rubber (mattresses and upholstery)
Stainproof upholstery and carpets
Synthetic clothing, fabric, sheets, and towels

Teflon pots and pans
Tin cans with phenol lining
Tobacco smoke
Toothpaste
Turpentine
Varnishes

Suggestions to Overcome Chemical Sensitivities

- Avoid the pollutant whenever possible.
- Use an air filter whenever possible.
- Drink filtered water and eat organic food.
- Use nutritional therapy including antioxidants.
- Begin allergy treatment.
- Boost your immune system and detoxify with nutritional supplements and herbs such as Vitamin C, E, selenium, zinc, glutathione, N–Acetyl cysteine, alpha–lipoic acid, silymarin (milk thistle) and red clover.

Are the Headaches You Get at Work Due to the Carpeting in Your Office?

The latest Environmental Protection Agency (EPA) studies have shown that despite the growing concern with outdoor air pollution, the level of indoor chemical pollution is generally higher than outdoor pollution. I have seen hundreds of patients who complain of an increase in their symptoms when they are indoors, especially if they have recently moved into a new home, changed schools, or have a new workplace. In this example, the chemicals found within these buildings may be triggering their symptoms. Your physician must take a very thorough history in helping to diagnose this problem. One of the clues that I often look for is whether or not your symptoms are better or worse on the days when you are in school or at work. If your symptoms are worse during these times, your indoor environment may be a contributing factor. The following table supplies vital information to help you identify your chemical irritants, and suggests some possible remedies.

COMMON INDOOR IRRITANTS

Pollutant	Source	Effects	Remedies
Tobacco smoke	Smoking.	Respiratory problems, cancer.	Ban smoking; ventilate home.
Radon	Natural radioactive gas enters through cracked foundations and along pipes.	Lung cancer; greatest risk to smokers.	Test home with charcoal canister or other simple detectors and use professional remediation if necessary.
Asbestos	Insulation on pipes and furnaces, floor and ceiling tiles.	Airborne fibers can cause cancer and other respiratory diseases.	Don't disturb suspected surfaces; contact professional for removal; service furnace.
Carbon monoxide	Blocked chimney or furnace flue, gas or kerosene space heaters, unvented gas stoves, seepage from garage.	Fatigue, headaches, unconsciousness, death.	Open windows; have appliances or chimney checked; install furnace draft fan to reduce exhaust back-draft risks.
Airborne lead paint	Paint removal, paint chips containing lead.	Poisoning, neurological damage, death.	Don't sand or burn off lead-based paint; wallpaper over flat surfaces; have professional replace woodwork.
Pesticides	Bug sprays and bombs, products applied by exterminators, pesticides on grains and produce.	Eye and respiratory irritation, damage to central nervous system and kidneys, cancer.	Increase ventilation; follow directions carefully; try nonchemical tactics, such as cleaning produce thoroughly.
Formaldehyde	Over 3,000 building products including plywood subflooring, wall paneling, cabinets, countertops, adhesives for carpeting, particleboard, linoleum, fiberboard, upholstery, and laminates.	Eye and respiratory irritation, headaches, nausea, rash, suspected cause of cancer.	Use "exterior-grade" pressed wood products; increase ventilation; cover affected surfaces with sealer; use plants such as philodendron and spider plants; use formaldehyde-free fiberboard underlay for countertops.

Pollutant	Source	Effects	Remedies
Paradichlorobenzene	Mothballs, air fresheners.	Respiratory irritant, causes cancer in animals.	Ventilate rooms; use cedar chips or sachets.
Perchloroethylene	Fumes from cleaning fluid residue in dry-cleaned clothes.	Dizziness, nausea, causes cancer in animals.	Air clothes before storing; switch to new dry cleaner if smell is strong.
Benzene, toluene, xylene, styrene	Tobacco smoke, stored fuels, solvents in oil-based paints and varnishes, auto exhaust, carpeting, padding, and backing.	Nausea, headache, dizziness, cancer; dust mites in carpeting cause allergic reactions and respiratory distress.	Ban smoking; ventilate home; dispose of unused paint and fuel; use natural paints made from plant resins, clay, and mineral pigments; use cotton and wool area rugs.
Chloroform	Chlorine in hot water for shower, washing machine.	Heavy exposure can increase cancer risk.	Install exhaust fan over shower; open windows.
Bacteria, fungi	Air conditioners, humidifiers.	Allergies, asthma, infectious diseases.	Change humidifier water daily; clean tank often; keep air conditioner filters clean.
Airborne particles	Wood stoves, fireplaces, tobacco smoke, ultrasonic humidifiers filled with tap water.	Respiratory problems; particles also carry radon and other pollutants into lungs.	Use wood stove with tight-fitting door; ventilate house; fill humidifier with distilled water; replace ultrasonic unit.
Vinyl chloride	Sheet flooring in kitchens and bathrooms, furniture coverings.	Ulcers, skin diseases, cancer, liver dysfunction.	Use ceramic tile or wood floor coverings; use natural fiber furniture coverings.

Indoor air pollution is one of the greatest health threats of all environmental problems. It ranks as the fourth highest cancer risk and poses the third greatest risk to human health.
—The Environmental Protection Agency (EPA)

What Are the Most Prevalent Chemical Irritants?

Formaldehyde, ethanol, phenol, glycerine, and petrochemicals are common irritants. They are found in large quantities throughout our workplace and home environments. If you develop a headache when traveling by air, it may be due to the ethanol in airport fumes. If you feel light-headed when cleaning the house, you may be having a reaction to the phenol in your disinfectant. If your eyes swell while applying makeup, it could be due to the glycerine in your cosmetics. Check the list below for sources of some of the most common chemical irritants.

SOURCES OF FOUR PREVALENT CHEMICAL IRRITANTS

Ethanol

Aftershave
Airport fumes
Asphalt
Cosmetics
Crude petroleum and its
    derivatives
Deodorant
Detergents
Disinfectants
Exhaust fumes
Gasoline
Glue
Hair spray
Insect spray
Mothballs
Paint
Perfumes
Shampoo
Shellac
Soaps
Varnish

Petrochemicals (Gas or Diesel)

Airport fumes
Car exhaust
Gas heat, stoves, or furnaces
Oil heat or furnaces

Phenol

Acne medications
Adhesives
Aspirin
Baking powders
Cosmetic preservatives in mascara,
    liquid eyeliner, cream rouges,
    and eye shadows
Detergents
Disinfectants
Dyes
Enamel paint
Epoxy
Explosives
Fiberglas
Flame retardant finishes
Food additives
Germicidal paints
Herbicides
Inks (fountain pens, printers)
Insulation (thermal and acoustical)
Jute/hemp fiber preservative
    (carpet backing, area rugs,
    rope, twine)
Laundry starches
Matches
Metal polishes
Mildew proofing
Nylon
Paint
Pesticides

Pharmaceuticals
Phenolic resins
Photographic chemicals
Plastics
Plywood
Preservatives in medications
    (allergy shots, nasal sprays,
    bronchial mists, cough syrups,
    eye drops, antihistamines, cold
    capsules, decongestants, first
    aid ointments)
Sealants
Shaving creams and lotions
Shoe polish
Solvents
Soundproofing
Spandex (girdles, support hose, etc.)
Stamp pads
Synthetic fibers
Tin can inner linings
Watercolor paints

Glycerine

Wood preservatives
Adhesives
Aftershave lotions
Antifreeze
Astringents
Cosmetics (especially in
    cakes or compacts)
Cough drops
Disinfectants
Dry-cleaning agents
Eye drops
Fabric softeners
Face masks
Fire retardant for textiles
Flavorings
Floor polishes
Food additives
Furniture polish
Inks
Latex paints
Leather
Liquid soaps
Margarines
Modeling clay
Mouthwashes
Nail polish
Oven cleaners
Paper
Perfume
Pharmaceuticals
Plastics
Polyurethane foam
Regenerated cellulose
Saddle soaps
Shaving creams and lotions
Shoe polishes
Shortenings
Solvents
Styptic pencils
Suntan preparations
Textile finishes
Toothpastes
Window cleaners

A Word about Formaldehyde

Formaldehyde is used in industrial chemicals and is becoming increasingly troublesome to sensitive individuals. There are numerous sources of formaldehyde with which we come in contact on a daily basis. Common names include formalin and methanol. Low-grade formaldehyde exposure is a primary cause of burning eyes, headaches, nasal irritation, and flu-like symptoms.

Uses of Formaldehyde

- Synthesis of alcohols, acids, and other chemicals
- Slow-release nitrogen fertilizers
- Concrete and plaster
- Antiperspirants
- Germicidal and detergent soaps
- Antiseptic in mouthwashes
- Shampoos
- Air deodorants
- Manufacture of antibiotics
- Disinfectant for sickrooms and surgical instruments
- Dyes and stripping agents
- Glues and adhesives
- Explosives
- Fireproofing substances applied to fabrics
- Insecticidal solutions for flies, mosquitoes, and moths
- Rodent poison
- Paper products
- Photographic developing solutions
- Component parts of wallboard and particleboard
- Resin in nail polish and undercoatings
- Plywood and pressboard (particularly in mobile homes)
- Waxes and polishes

TIPS

For healthier air travel:
- Bring your own fresh food and beverages.
- Before traveling, soak in an electrolyte bath of Epsom salts, cider vinegar, and baking soda.
- Drink plenty of liquids such as club soda, bottled water, or apple juice during the flight.

Can Common Houseplants Conquer Your Pollution Problems?

Since plants breathe in carbon dioxide and exhale oxygen, they may be effective in removing pollutants from the air. The Foliage for Clean Air Council (FCAC) has published the following information regarding plants and their protection against pollution based on twenty years of study by the National Aeronautics & Space Administration (NASA). The FCAC advises using one potted plant per 100 square feet of floor area to remove airborne pollutants.

Keep in mind, however, that if you are extremely mold-sensitive, indoor plants should probably be avoided.

PLANT SOLUTIONS TO POLLUTION

Pollutant	Sources	Health Risks	Removed by
Formaldehyde	Foam insulation Plywood Particleboard Fire retardant on clothing or fabric Paneling Glues and adhesives Paint Mobile homes Carpeting Furniture Paper goods Household cleaners Water repellents Air deodorizers Insecticides	Headaches Eye irritation Upper respiratory distress Asthma Throat cancer	Philodendron Spider plant Golden pathos Corn plant Chrysanthemum Mother-in-law's tongue Azalea Dieffenbachia Bamboo palm
Benzene	Tobacco smoke Gasoline Synthetic fibers Plastics Inks Oils Detergents Rubber	Skin irritation Eye irritation Headaches Loss of appetite Drowsiness Leukemia and blood diseases	English ivy Marginata Janet craig Chrysanthemum Gerbera daisy Warneckei Peace lily
Trichloroethylene	Paints Varnishes Lacquers Adhesives Inks Dry cleaning	Liver cancer	Gerbera daisy Chrysanthemum Peace lily Warneckei Marginata

Could Your Child's Learning Disabilities Be Due to Lead Toxicity?

With each passing year, I see a larger number of patients who, unfortunately, have high levels of toxic metals in their body. Heavy metal toxicity is an increasingly troublesome problem in our society. Each year, more and more toxic metals are found in our food and water supply, in industrial pollutants, in household products, and in various other sources. Metals can have adverse effects on various parts of your body, including the brain, liver, muscles, and kidneys. Heavy metals can accumulate in your body over time, inhibiting your enzyme systems and metabolic processes, thereby contributing to many of your health problems.

EFFECTS OF TOXIC METALS ON BODY

SOURCES OF TOXIC METALS		TARGET TISSUES	SYMPTOMS
Aluminum • Antacids • Deodorants • Cooking utensils • Table salt	• Cans • Aluminum cookware • Aluminum foil	Central nervous system	May possibly lead to Alzheimer's disease
Arsenic • Pesticide residue • Rat poison • Seafood • Automotive exhaust • Soil	• Paper • Paint • Ceramics • Glass	Skin Muscles Peripheral nerves	Drowsiness Confusion Weakness Muscle aches
Cadmium • Cigarette smoke • Oysters • Paints • Metals	• Antiseptics • Fertilizers	Liver Kidneys	Abdominal cramps Headaches Hypertension Nausea Vomiting
Lead • Drinking water • Canned foods • Newsprint • Plaster • Gasoline • Pencils • Ceramics	• Airplane exhaust • Asphalt • Leaded paint • Welding • Dyes • Batteries • Auto exhaust	Kidneys Placenta Heart Bones Central nervous system	Anemia Dementia Learning disabilities

SOURCES OF TOXIC METALS		TARGET TISSUES	SYMPTOMS
Mercury		Central nervous system	Depression
• Fish	• Fungicides	Kidneys	Diarrhea
• Dental amalgams	• Floor polish	Liver	Fatigue
• Mercurochrome	• Adhesives		Insomnia or drowsiness
• Antiseptic	• Tattooing		Irritability
			Loss of memory
			Moodiness
			Nausea
			Senile dementia
			Stomatitis
			Tremors
			Vertigo
Nickel		Central nervous system	Anemia
• Glass and ceramics	• Electrical devices	Brain	Cancer
• Tobacco smoke	• Hydrogenated oils	Heart	Heart attack
• Steel and metal alloys			Lung hemorrhages

Lead exposure can impair physical and mental development, cause central nervous system damage, and even lead to death.

—Centers for Disease Control

Did You Know That Vitamin and Mineral Deficiencies Can Make You More Susceptible to the Adverse Effects of Chemicals?

A deficiency in specific vitamins, trace minerals, or other vital nutrients can make you more susceptible to the adverse effects of various environmental chemicals or toxic metals. Optimizing your nutrient intake and preventing deficiencies are thus paramount to help your immune system withstand the effects of environmental chemicals. For example, if you are deficient in zinc, you will be more susceptible to the adverse effects of the heavy metal cadmium. Similarly, if you are low in vitamin C, you can become prone to the ill effects of lead exposure. Many of the vitamins and minerals listed below function as important antioxidants and are crucial for normal metabolism, detoxification, and cellular function.

If You Are Deficient in the Following Nutrients:	You May Be Susceptible to the Adverse Effects of:
Vitamin A	DDT, hydrocarbon carcinogens, PCBs
Vitamin C	Arsenic, cadmium, carbon monoxide, chromium, DDT, dieldrin, lead, mercury, nitrates, ozone
Vitamin E	Lead, ozone
Calcium	Lead
Iron	Hydrocarbon carcinogens, lead, manganese
Magnesium	Fluoride
Phosphorus	Lead
Protein	DDT, other insecticides
Riboflavin	Hydrocarbon carcinogens, lead, ozone
Selenium	Cadmium, mercury, ozone
Zinc	Cadmium

TIPS

Assist in chemical detoxification by:
- Adding antioxidant supplements such as selenium, vitamins A, C, and E, methionine, cysteine, glutathione, alpha–lipoic acid, zinc and beta-carotene to your daily program.
- Soaking in an electrolyte bath of Epsom salt, cider vinegar, and baking soda.
- Keep your bowels moving by adding more fiber to your diet.
- Assist liver detoxification by drinking the juice made from a mixture of carrots, celery, beets, and parsley along with the herbs milk thistle and red clover.

CHAPTER 15

Safer Alternatives

While millions of dollars continue to be poured into cancer research, there are others of us who believe that the most effective research is that done by the individual as he examines his own eating and living habits.

— Richard O. Brennan, M.D.

As more chemicals are continually being poured into our food supply, cosmetics, soaps, detergents, personal products, cleaning agents, and insecticides and pesticides, it is increasingly important to look for less chemically contaminated, environmentally friendly and hypoallergenic products. As the public demand increases, the number of safer alternatives and hypoallergenic products to reach the marketplace will continue to grow. I have treated hundreds of chemically sensitive patients over the years who have had to make significant changes in their lifestyle and selection of personal products and cleaning agents. This chapter will provide you with some of the options that I have found to be most useful.

Personal Products: Are There Safer Alternatives?

Fortunately, manufacturers of cosmetics, toiletries, and personal products are becoming more environmentally conscientious and manufacturing safer products. More importantly, however, is the fact that the public continues to demand safer and less odorous deodorants, shampoos, toothpastes, and other cosmetic products. If you are chemically sensitive or if you're simply looking for more environmentally friendly choices for personal products, the following list of substitutions may be helpful.

PERSONAL PRODUCT ALTERNATIVES

Product	Substitution
Cosmetics	Purchase 100% fragrance-free, allergy-tested products such as Clinique, Almay, Gabriel, and Ecco Bella. Try individualized formulations.
Dandruff treatment	Home Health Everclean or tea tree oil shampoo. Try ½ cup lemon juice + 1 cup water. Try ½ cup apple cider vinegar + ½ cup water. Apply directly to scalp before shampooing. Rinse hair with solution of Zephiran (½ tsp per cup water).
Deodorant	Dab damp washcloth in baking soda or apply with damp cotton ball. Look for aluminum-free products manufactured by companies such as Desert Essence, Jason, Weleda, Mill Creek, Tom's of Maine, and Aubrey Organics.
Hair color	Use natural color from henna and plant-based extracts. Look for products by Rainbow, NaturColor, Vitawave, or Light Mountain.
Hair rinse	Use baking soda or vinegar to neutralize chemicals. Look for products by Ecco Bella, Nature's Gate, and Shi-Kai.
Moisturizer	Try almond oil, vegetable oil, apricot oil, jojoba, or coconut oil. An abundance of natural products are available. Suggested brands include Nature's Gate, Kiss My Face, and Alba Botanica.
Mouthwash	Use baking soda in water. Look for alcohol-free products from Tom's of Maine and Desert Essence.
Permanents	Try Ogilvie Act I, which has no strong odors, Rave, which has no ammonia, or Vitawave.
Shampoo	Look for unscented products that don't contain DEA, formaldehyde, or coloring. Many products are available at your health food market. Look for Nature's Gate, Aubrey Organics, Shi-Kai, Tom's of Maine, or Ecco Bella.
Shaving cream	Try Neo-Life Green, Kiss My Face, Tom's of Maine, or Alba Botanica.
Soap	Try Basis, Unscented Neutrogena, Ivory, Dr. Bronner's, Kiss My Face, Simple Soap, Pure Castille, Rokeach, Bon Ami Cake, or Pure Olive Soap.
Tissues—toilet and facial (white only)	Try Seventh Generation, Banner, Scott tissue, or Kleenex regular.
Toothpaste	Use baking soda and/or sea salt. Look for Tom's of Maine, Nature's Gate, Peela, or Desert Essence products.

TIP

• If you are excessively sensitive to the odors from personal products or cleaning agents, you might find it helpful to purchase a charcoal face mask to help avoid inhaling the noxious fumes.

Do You Feel Sick from Your Cleaning Agents?

Household cleaning products represent a major source of chemical pollution. If you are chemically sensitive, or simply trying to be environmentally conscientious, you should do your best to avoid synthetic chemicals. Try to substitute safer cleaning agents in place of those containing potentially toxic chemicals. Fortunately, there are more safer cleaning products on the market than ever before. Look for products that are hypoallergenic, without petroleum, phosphates, or other harsh chemicals. You can usually find these products either through an independent distributor or at your local health food store. Some of these cleaning agents can also be found at your local grocery store.

SAFER ALTERNATIVES AS CLEANING AGENTS

Avoid	Use
All-purpose heavy-duty cleaners that contain hydrocarbons such as benzene	Amway LOC, Shaklee Basic H, Trisodium Phosphate (TSP) (available at hardware stores), Neo-Life, Simple Green, Seventh Generation, Bon Ami, Zephiran chloride, or Borax
Chemical neutralizers (products that remove scents)	Put ½ cup of dry baking soda in a container or use a molecular absorber by Abzorbstar.
Chrome cleaners that contain ammonia, ethanol, fragrances, or petroleum distillates	Pure cider vinegar applied with soft cloth and buffed with paper towel; Whiting (calcium carbonate) available at paint stores
Dishwashing compounds containing perfume, hydrocarbons, or formaldehyde	Shaklee Basic D, Amway Dishdrops, Neo-Life, Seventh Generation
Disinfectants containing ammonia or phenol	Borax, Shaklee, or Amway products or Seventh Generation
Fabric softeners containing perfumes or hydrocarbons	Calgon or add ½ cup of vinegar to rinse water
Furniture polish containing fragrances, ammonia, or petroleum distillates	Murphy's Oil Soap, Beeswax, 100% pure olive oil, or lemon oil
House paint that contains formaldehyde, ammonia, lead, or volatile hydrocarbons	Try brands such as AFM, Glidden 2000, Benjamin Moore, Sears 840 Series, Miller, or other latex pains without fungicides or biocides. You also might want to add two to three tablespoons of baking soda to each gallon of paint to reduce the odor.
Laundry bleach containing chlorine	Hydrogen peroxide (add ½ cup to washing machine), Clorox II, Snowy Bleach, Borax-20 Mule Team, Borateem Bleach, or sodium percarbonate from Ecover.
Laundry detergent containing perfume, formaldehyde, or alcohol	Shaklee Basic L, Amway SA8, Neo-Life, Unscented Tide, Ivory Detergent, Simple Green, Seventh Generation, Borax, or Ecover
Laundry whitener	Borax-20 Mule Team, Miracle White
Mold inhibitors containing formaldehyde, chlorine, or hydrocarbons	Tea Tree Oil by Desert Essence, Borax powder, lemon juice, or zephiran chloride 17% (mix 1 oz per gallon of water)

Avoid	Use
Room deodorizers containing perfumes, alcohol, or petroleum distillates	Borax, baking soda, Tea Tree Oil by Desert Essence, 1–2 tablespoons of vanilla extract in a small cup, or use an electric fan to blow air out of a musty or stale-smelling room
Scouring powders that contain chlorine and hydrocarbons	Bon Ami, Borax, baking soda
Shoe polish	Use cooking oils, small amounts of olive or lemon oil; buff with soft cloth.
Stain removers that contain chlorine, formaldehyde, toluene, or benzene	Hydrogen peroxide, lemon juice mixed with sea salt, Neo-Life Rugged Red, or Borax
Sterling silver cleaner that contains fragrances, ammonia, and petroleum distillates	Whiting on damp cloth or soapy solution of baking soda and water
Window cleaners containing ammonia	Borax, baking soda and water, Bon Ami cake soap, or Zephiran chloride

The above alternatives may not be tolerated by everyone but have been found to be much better tolerated by most people. Furthermore, they are much safer for the environment as they generally cause less pollution. There are also an abundance of new and healthy household products that are continually being added to the marketplace and are becoming readily available. Look for products manufactured by Seventh Generation, Bon Ami, Earth Friendly Products, Ecover, Murphy's, and AFM.

Should I Use a Water Filter?

You may want to consider purchasing a water purification system for your home since tap water is frequently contaminated with organic hydrocarbons such as trichloroethane, toluene, benzene, and trihalomethane. You can look either for a model that sits on top of the sink, one that is installed under the sink, or perhaps a central filter that purifies all the water throughout your home. If necessary, you can also purchase a water filter that is attached to your shower head to specifically filter your bathing water. I have found this to be particularly useful if you experience skin redness, itching, or hives after taking a shower. A water filter can also help to eliminate contamination problems including parasites, lead, chlorine, bacteria, bad taste, and foul-smelling odors.

You may purchase either spring or distilled water, and when possible, choose water supplied in glass containers. If water sits in a plastic container for a long time, some of the plasticizers can leach out into the water. There are three main water purification systems for your home: carbon block, distillation, or reverse osmosis. I have used a carbon filter in my home for more than ten years and have found it to improve the taste and healthfulness of my water. I have found the following brands of filters to be particularly effective: Daulton, Elite, Seagull, and Water Cleen. The following table gives an overview of the three main types of purification systems readily available.

WATER PURIFICATION SYSTEMS

Purification Through Carbon Block

This form of filtration is the most practical, inexpensive, and popular for residential use. However, the filters must be changed regularly to prevent bacteria from breeding or mold growth in the carbon medium. It also is effective in removing the bad taste or odor that may be found in your drinking water.

Removes	Does Not Remove
Bacteria	Fluoride
Chlorine	Heavy metals
Chloroform	Minerals
Organic chemicals	Nitrates
Pesticides	Salts

Purification Through Distillation

This is probably the most expensive form of water purification. Since these units tend to build up sediment on a regular basis, you have to remove it periodically.

Removes	Does Not Remove
Asbestos	Chlorine
Bacteria	Organic chemicals
Fluorides	
Heavy metals	
Minerals	
Nitrates	
Salts	
Viruses	

Purification Through Reverse Osmosis

In this case, three filters are arranged in a series. They include a sediment filter, a reverse osmosis filter, and an activated carbon cartridge.

Removes	Does Not Remove
Asbestos	Bacteria
Chlorine compounds	Chemicals
Fluorides	Chlorine
Heavy metals	Minerals
Large particulate matter	Pesticides
Most organic chemicals and pesticides	Viruses
Nitrates	

Getting the Bugs Out Naturally!

We have all probably been exposed to insecticides at some time in our lives. For example, you may have had the exterminator come to your house on a monthly basis to keep those little critters from finding their way onto your bathroom floor. Even though you may not have noted an objectionable smell, insecticides still have potentially damaging short- and long-term effects on your body. These poisonous chemicals may cause headaches, dizziness, rashes and shortness of breath, as well as cancer and other chronic illnesses. Chemicals may enter your body by inhalation, ingestion, or absorption through the skin. Because insecticides are often used in the home, school, or workplace, it is important that you limit your exposure to them whenever you can. The following table provides some safer alternatives for insect control. They don't work 100 percent of the time, but it is certainly worth giving them a try.

Roaches

Meticulous Cleaning
- Minimize crumbs.
- Store food in tightly sealed containers.
- Remove dirty dishes from sink.
- Keep sinks, tub, and showers dry.

Harris Roach Tablets
(Keep away from children and pets.)
- Purchase at grocery stores.

Boric Acid Powder
- Sprinkle or mix with water (50% concentration). Spray liberally into crevices, corners, moldings.

Diatomaceous Earth
(obstructs insect's breathing apparatus)
- Purchase at swimming pool supply stores.

One Part Plaster of Paris to One Part Flour
- Was used during World War I

Roach Candy
- Mix 16 oz powdered boric acid, 1 cup flour, ¼ cup sugar, 1 small chopped onion (optional), ½ cup shortening (or 70% flour, 10% sugar, 10% cocoa powder, 10% boric acid, or borax).
- Shape into small balls.
- Place throughout house.
- Keep away from children or pets.
- Discard when dry.

Baking Soda Mixed with Powdered Sugar
- Sprinkle mixture.

Fleas

Wash Pets and Bedding
- While fleas are still waterlogged and slow, use tweezers to pick off.

Natural Flea Collars
- Use herbs available at health food stores to repel fleas.

Brewer's Yeast
- Feed to pets.
- Vitamin B_1 in the yeast produces an odor that repels fleas.

Pennyroyal, Sassafras, Camellia, or Eucalyptus
- Mix with oils.
- Use in cracks and crevices where fleas lay eggs.

Pennyroyal or Eucalyptus Oil
- Soak rope in oil and place around your pet's neck.

Diatomaceous Earth
- Purchase at swimming pool supply stores.

Drown Fleas
- Remove all pets from room.
- Place shallow dish of water containing dishwashing detergent on floor.

Ants and Crickets

Cleanliness
- Minimize crumbs.
- Seal food containers tightly.
- Clean sink.
- Minimize sources of food and water.

Powdered Red Chili Pepper, Paprika, Dried Peppermint
- Sprinkle mixture.

Borax Powder or Boric Acid Powder
- Add to bait such substances as powdered sugar, flour, and cocoa. You will need at least 40 percent concentration for toxicity. Make sure you keep children and pets away.

Boric Acid Powder
- Mix with mashed potatoes or honey.

Castor Oil
- Cover holes, cracks, seams.

Tansey Herb Tea
- Make tea. Spray around house.

Ticks

Tincture of Merthiolate
- Ticks will loosen hold if touched by a drop of merthiolate or with a hot match. You can then pull it off with tweezers.

Flies

Fly Paper
- Make paper by boiling sugar, corn syrup and water, and placing mixture on brown paper strips.

- Fly Swatter

Moths

Mothball Alternative
- Kill eggs by placing items in sun or run through warm dryer.
- Store items in clean airtight containers.

Sachets
- Make cotton, linen, or silk sachets filled with dried lavender or equal parts of dried rosemary, mint, thyme, ginseng, and 2 tablespoons of cloves.
- Place in drawers and closets.

Dried Tobacco
- Put in closets or chests.

Whole Peppercorns, Cedar Oil, or Cedar Chips
- Put in closets or chests.

Rats and Rodents

Traps
- Bait with cheese, bacon, or chocolate.

Plaster of Paris
- Mix 25–50% plaster of paris with flour, sugar, and cocoa. Poses little hazard to children or pets.

Cleanliness
- Minimize crumbs.

Steel Wool
- Plug points of entry to shut off food supply.

Cornmeal/Warfarin
- Prepare bait of 10–20 parts fresh corn meal to 1 part warfarin. This is a prescription drug commonly used as a blood thinner. Keep children and pets away from this mixture.

Part IV

LIFESTYLE MODIFICATIONS

CHAPTER 16

Enthusiastic Exercise Enhances Endurance

It is much cheaper and more effective to maintain good health than it is to regain it once it is lost.
—Kenneth H. Cooper, M.D., M.P.H.

Exercising regularly should be a part of everyday life. Varying your exercise routine provides maximum benefit and enhances enjoyment. It is important to combine aerobic exercise such as jogging, bicycling, and swimming with anaerobic activities such as weight lifting and stretching.

What Are the Benefits of Exercise?

Exercise:

- Reduces the risk of diabetes by improving glucose utilization.
- Promotes blood circulation.
- Increases oxygen intake.
- Burns calories and promotes weight loss.
- Boosts energy and endurance.
- Brings blood pressure down.
- Prevents bone loss.
- Strengthens the heart.

- Relieves stress.
- Lowers cholesterol.
- Reduces the risk of heart disease.
- Improves strength, range of motion, and flexibility.
- Helps to prevent injury.
- Increases self-esteem.
- May have anti-aging effects.
- Keeps your mind sharper.

Comparative Benefits of Exercise (rated on a scale of 0–100)

	Running	Bicycling	Swimming	Handball	Tennis	Walking	Golf	Bowling
Cardiorespiratory endurance	100	90	100	90	76	62	38	24
Muscular endurance	95	86	95	86	76	67	38	2
Strength	81	76	67	71	67	52	43	24
Flexibility	43	43	71	76	67	33	38	33
Balance	81	86	57	81	76	38	38	29
Weight control	100	95	71	90	76	62	29	24
Muscle definition	67	71	67	52	62	52	29	24
Digestion	62	57	62	62	57	52	33	33
Sleep	76	71	76	57	52	67	29	29

TIPS

- Do 20–30 minutes of continuous exercise 3–4 times per week.
- Try to maintain your pulse rate within your target zone, as discussed on page 187.

How Many Calories Do You Burn Doing Housework?

Each exercise activity burns calories at a different rate. You should vary your routine to maximize your enjoyment while toning and strengthening different muscle groups. The table below approximates the number of calories burned per hour of activity.

ACTIVITY RECOMMENDATIONS

Activity	Approximate Calories Burned per Hour	Activity	Approximate Calories Burned per Hour
Backpacking, hiking	450–500	Jogging (10 min/mi)	550–650
Baseball, softball	250–350	Judo, karate	250–300
Basketball	350–400	Manual labor	450–500
Bicycling (5.5 mph)	200–350	Rope jumping	750–850
Bicycling (13 mph)	600–650	Rowing machine	550–650
Bowling	250–300	Running (7.5 min/mi)	750–850
Calisthenics	250–300	Running in place	600–700
Chopping wood	250–300	Shoveling	350–400
Dancing, fast	350–400	Skating	300–450
Dancing, slow	250–300	Skiing (cross–country)	1,200
Football	300–400	Swimming (25 yd/min)	250–300
Gardening (light)	250–300	Tennis—singles	350–450
Golfing	250–300	Walking (2 mph)	200–280
Horseback riding	250–400	Walking (4½ mph)	400–480
Housework	250–300		

What Should Your Pulse Rate Be During Exercise?

While engaged in an exercise activity, you should strive to maintain your pulse rate within your target zone. Your target zone is based on your age and your physical condition. If you are taking prescription medication, especially those that affect your heart rate, your target zone may be less than the chart below. Check with your doctor before beginning any exercise program.

To take your pulse:
• Lightly place two fingertips on the main artery in your neck.
• Count your pulse for 15 seconds, beginning with 0. Multiply by 4.
• This will give you your pulse rate per minute.

TARGET ZONE

Age	15	20	25	30	35	40	45	50	55	60	65	70
Minimum Heart Rate	140	140	136	133	130	126	122	119	115	112	108	105
Maximum Heart Rate	160	160	156	152	148	144	140	136	132	128	124	120

Why Is Stretching Important?

Stretching is essential to avoid injury and muscle cramps. Stretching increases your flexibility and range of motion, strengthens a weak back, and alleviates lower back pain. To help reduce risk of injury, it is always a good idea to stretch before doing any strenuous exercise and for a few minutes after exercise. The following is a simple stretch routine you can do every day. Remember to breathe deeply. Try to hold each position for a minimum of five seconds, and work your way up to thirty seconds. Repeat each stretch a minimum of three times. Never force a stretch. Stretching should be done slowly and gently. If you have had any recent surgery, muscle or joint problems, please consult your physician or a health-care professional before starting this stretching program.

STRETCHES

Head, Neck, and Shoulders
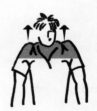

- Raise top of shoulders toward ears, hold and then release.
- Turn head toward right shoulder and then toward left shoulder, then drop chin to chest.
- Hold each position 3–5 seconds and release.
- Repeat each of these 3–5 times.

Chest
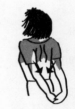

- Clasp hands behind back. Try to straighten elbows and rotate shoulders back. Pull clasped hand upward.
- Variation 1: Place palms together. Hold at heart level. Press hands together.

Legs
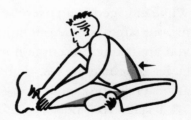

- Sit on floor with one leg extended and one foot flexed.
- Bend the other leg with heel to groin.
- Bend over toward flexed foot and hold there for 5 seconds. Work up to 30 seconds.
- Repeat on other side.
- Variation 1: Standing, reach with left hand overhead stretching one side toward left foot then repeat on opposite side.
- Variation 2: Standing, reach for ankle and then toes, pressing head to knees.
- Hold 5–30 seconds.

Groin
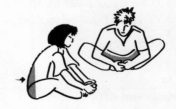

- Sit on floor and bring soles of feet together.
- Gently push the knees toward the floor sitting up straight.
- Hold 5–30 seconds and repeat three times.

Back and Lymphatic System

- Lie on back and pull one knee to your chest and hold.
- Extend leg straight up, flex foot, and hold 3–5 seconds.
- With leg extended, rotate ankle to the left and then to the right five times in each direction.
- Repeat three times on each leg.

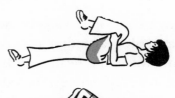

Triceps

- Extend right arm upward, hold elbow to ear, and bend arm.
- With left hand, gently pull elbow left toward ear.
- Repeat three times with both right and left arm.

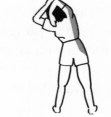

Hip and Lower Back

- Lie on your back with right leg extended.
- Bend left leg and cross it over the right leg.
- Extend right arm and turn head to follow right arm.
- With left hand, gently coax right knee to floor.
- Repeat with left leg extended.

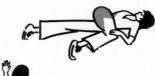

Thighs

- Stand facing wall, leaning on wall with left hand for balance.
- With right hand, hold top of left foot.
- Gently pull heel toward buttocks.
- Repeat with opposite hand to opposite foot.

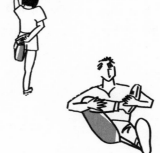

Hips and Hamstrings

- Sit against wall with left leg extended.
- With left hand clasped outside of right ankle.
- Bend right knee and gently pull toward chest.
- Repeat with right hand and left ankle.

Achilles Tendon and Calves

- Stand facing wall.
- Bend right knee and place in front of left leg, approximately one foot apart.
- Move hips toward wall until a stretch is felt in calf, supporting yourself by leaning on the wall.
- Keep heels on floor and hold for 30 seconds.
- Repeat on the other side.

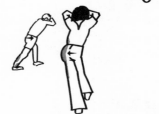

Back

- Lie on stomach with arms and legs extended.
- Raise right arm and left leg, keeping head up.
- Repeat with left arm and right leg three times each.

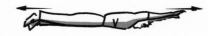

Spine

- Lie on back.
- Pull both legs to chest. Slowly bring head, neck, and shoulders forward and tighten stomach.

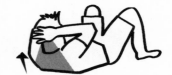

What Are the Benefits of Walking?

Many people find walking the easiest and most satisfying of all exercises. It can be performed all year round at virtually no cost. Walking has been shown to improve circulation, protect the heart, and boost the immune system. It can also help to prevent bone loss, assist in keeping your bowels more regular, and put you in a better frame of mind.

Walking at a brisk pace for a sufficient period of time to stimulate the heart, lungs, and circulatory system provides long-term benefits and makes a good transition to get into shape before beginning other more strenuous physical activities.

To get started on a walking program, begin walking fifteen minutes per day, four days per week. Gradually build up to a minimum of thirty minutes per day, five days per week. Check to make sure your heart rate is within your target zone as discussed previously on page 185. Remember to stretch before and after walking. You may enjoy walking more by having a partner join you.

Make sure you have comfortably fitting walking shoes or sneakers and that you are dressed appropriately. I find it to be invigorating to take a brisk walk in the morning before starting the rest of my day. In addition, I find that taking a walk after work can also alleviate a lot of stress, reduce fatigue, and boost energy.

Part V

PROGRESSIVE HEALING TECHNIQUES

CHAPTER 17

Mind-Body Connection

*The universe is full of magical things, patiently waiting for
our wits to grow sharper.*

—Bertrand Russell

Your thought processes play a vital role in health and disease. Maintaining a positive attitude assists your immune system by aiding in the production of neurotransmitters and other naturally occuring substances known as mediators and cytokines. These substances play an integral part in the healing process and play a role in relieving pain through the secretion of endorphins. Your thought processes also have a profound effect on reducing stress and making you feel more at ease with yourself and those around you. By getting involved in stress reduction techniques, you will be able to oxygenate your tissues more effectively and improve circulation. Try spending at least ten minutes each day using some of the relaxation techniques discussed in this chapter.

The following modalities have been found to be effective in lowering blood pressure, alleviating headaches, reducing stress and achieving better health. If necessary, consider taking a class or meeting with a counselor or therapist who can assist you in integrating these modalities into your life.

Relaxation Therapies

Relaxation therapies include yoga, biofeedback, guided imagery, and meditation. Deep relaxation has been found to improve immune response, reduce stress, alleviate headaches, lower blood pressure, and treat coronary heart disease.

You may want to try starting a relaxation technique by simply sitting comfortably on the floor or in a chair in a quiet room. Pick a pleasant word or term to focus on and begin taking deep, slow breaths with your eyes closed and muscles relaxed. As you exhale, silently focus on the word that you chose. In time, you will be able to disconnect your thoughts of work, family, or other thoughts that come into your mind. Try to do this exercise for at least ten minutes per day. You will generally feel much more relaxed and uplifted for the remainder of the day.

Yoga

Yoga is a technique utilizing a variety of stretches and breathing exercises to unite the physical, mental, and spiritual energies of the mind and body. The practice of yoga has been shown to promote relaxation, health, and general vitality. Stress reduction, regulation of heart rate and blood pressure, improved muscle tone and flexibility, and slowing down the aging process are some of the benefits associated with yoga. I have also seen patients who experience fewer back or neck problems, have less painful joints associated with arthritis, suffer fewer asthma attacks, and experience less stress and more vitality during pregnancy if they practice yoga.

You may want to consider initially getting involved in a yoga class to teach you the different poses. From there, you can usually continue these on your own. I have also found it beneficial to watch videotapes of yoga while I perform the different movements.

Biofeedback

Biofeedback involves the use of electronic devices to control many bodily functions such as digestive processes, pulse and heart rate, skin temperature, circulation, and muscle and neurological function. Biofeedback can teach you how to promote wellness by consciously regulating these vital processes, which are normally perceived of as subconscious functions. Biofeedback may be useful in regulating blood pressure, reducing stress, relieving headaches, relieving muscle spasms, alleviating pain, and helping with sleep and gastrointestinal disorders. I have found biofeedback to be particularly helpful in patients with anxiety, panic attacks, insomnia, cold extremities, headaches, and in children with attention deficit disorder.

Guided Imagery

Guided imagery or visualization involves tapping the power of the mind by imagining pleasant sensations, thoughts, and ideas to beneficially affect your body and your emotional outlook. For example, if you are a dancer, you may imagine yourself on a stage and going through the entire repertoire of your performance in your mind. A basketball player may imagine himself shooting the winning basket with one second left in the game. These mental exercises generally help to improve self-confidence, concentration, and performance. Other benefits include slowing the heart rate, enhancing the immune system, reducing stress and high blood pressure, alleviating pain, controlling symptoms associated with PMS, and reducing stress-related gastrointestinal problems.

Meditation

There are various approaches to meditation. Some concentrate on the breath, an image, or a word, while other approaches expand the attention to the flow of thoughts, feelings, and sounds. Benefits of meditation include lower blood pressure, reduced stress and tension, decreased heart and pulse rate, enhanced immune response, increased circulation and oxygen consumption, and pain management. Getting involved in meditation can help you with self-confidence, concentration, and can simply give you an uplifting feeling and more vitality.

Acupuncture and Shiatzu

Acupuncture originated in China nearly 5,000 years ago. It involves the use of needles applied to specific points of the body to help revitalize or unblock the life force or energy flow, commonly known as Qi. Acupuncture is rapidly becoming more popular in the United States and other countries worldwide. It has been particularly useful in the treatment of chronic pain and can help reduce the necessity for medications. It also may be useful to help reduce dental pain especially after dental surgery or tooth extraction. Others find that acupuncture is useful if they are experiencing nausea from chemotherapy, morning sickness from pregnancy, or after undergoing surgical anesthesia. I have found that acupuncture may help my patients reduce their symptoms of depression, stress, tension headaches, insomnia, asthma, and arthritis.

If you are too squeamish to undergo acupunture with needles, there is always an alternative. You might find that a form of acupressure, known as shiatzu, is more suitable. Shiatzu involves the application of finger pressure to specific points on the body in a firm, rhythmic sequence to awaken acupuncture meridians. Some practitioners of shiatzu use their feet to apply the pressure to different points along the meridians. Shiatzu may help to reduce pain, increase circulation, alleviate headaches or nausea, help with menstrual cramps, and relieve gastrointestinal distress such as indigestion, heartburn, or constipation.

Massage

Virtually everyone would probably like to receive a massage on an occasional basis. Massage involves pressing, stroking, or manipulating your muscles and skin to improve the flow of energy, blood, and lymph. A massage can be very relaxing, soothing, stress-reducing, pain-relieving, and may even help to improve circulation, immune response, digestive difficulties, sport injuries, headaches, and chronic pain. Massage can be performed on virtually anyone including babies, the elderly, and even pregnant women before, during, or after childbirth.

Bodywork

There are a variety of different techniques which should probably come under the umbrella of the term "Bodywork." They are all designed to improve your flexibility, increase your range of motion, and allow your body to move more easily and freely. Bodywork techniques require hands-on manipulation of your muscles by a skilled practitioner. On the other hand, techniques involving energy medicine may not require hands-on treatment and may not involve any touching at all. This form of healing is still very controversial. Energy methods are thought to release blocked energy and to restore normal body functioning. The following is a brief discussion of some of the most common forms of bodywork:

Rolfing

Rolfing involves a deep tissue massage whose goal is to realign and balance your body. It is thought to improve posture and body alignment. The practitioner of Rolfing may use a variety of his or her body parts to perform the deep massage. This can include the hands, thumbs, knuckles, or even elbows and knees. Rolfing is thought to help with sports injuries, poor posture, flexibility, and maybe even breathing problems and anxiety.

Alexander Technique

The Alexander Technique was developed more than one hundred years ago and is also one that emphasizes the importance of improving your posture, body mechanics, range of motion, balance, and coordination. Its goal is to reverse muscle misuses that you have developed over the years. It teaches you how to stand and sit properly to help relieve stress and pressure from your head, neck, and other joints. The Alexander Technique has been useful for people suffering with chronic pain, arthritis, head, neck or spine injuries, and to simply remove stress and tension on your body. Incidentally, the Alexander Technique was my first introduction to alternative healing techniques in my early teenage years.

The Feldenkrais Method

The Feldenkrais Method combines movement training along with gentle touch in an effort to improve your coordination, flexibility, and range of motion. Your practitioner usually guides you through a series of movements while you are either sitting or standing.

There is certainly some overlap in many of the therapies which were just discussed. Many of these treatments are done in a group setting while others can be performed on an individual basis. I have found that it is frequently useful to try one of these mind-body techniques first in a group setting, if applicable, and then to practice it on your own for a time. You might find that one or more of these methods is more suitable for you than the others. In order to find a well-qualified and skilled health-care practioner in these fields, you might want to:

- Talk to a friend, neighbor, or open-minded physician and ask for a recommendation.
- Inquire at your local health food store. They are frequently good sources of information and may have a schedule of upcoming community lectures or seminars on a topic that you desire.
- Contact one of the national organizations that trains, licenses, or certifies practitioners of holistic medicine. In Appendix III, on pages 314–316, you will find the names and addresses of several national organizations that may be able to give you a recommendation for practitioners in your area.

> *The greatest discovery of any generation is that human beings can alter their lives by altering the attitudes of their minds.*
>
> —Albert Schweitzer

CHAPTER 18

Medicinal Herbs and Botanicals

Medicinal herbs are being used by an ever-increasing number of individuals to treat many common health complaints. Herbs are ingested as food, used as spices, and have been used as medicinal cures throughout history. Many herbs are commonly used in our pharmaceutical industry today and are components of prescription medication.

Herbs are becoming increasingly popular throughout the entire world. I have found that herbs can be effective in treating some of the most common problems that my patients complain of in a family practice setting. For example, feverfew can help relieve chronic headaches, aloe vera can be applied topically to accelerate the healing of burns or wounds, and garlic can help treat high blood pressure. At the same time, St. John's wort can be an effective antidepressant, green tea is a potent antioxidant, hawthorn can reduce angina pectoris, and milk thistle can effectively improve liver function. Herbs can be purchased in a variety of forms; fresh from the market, crushed in a capsule, mixed in a tincture, or served as a tea. Some herbs, however, such as black cohosh, St. John's wort, and kava kava should be puchased only in the "standard extract" form, which helps to ensure their potency and quality. In many instances, herbs can often be used as an alternative to prescription or over-the-counter medication. The following table provides a general overview of some of the main functions of the herbs I commonly recommend.

What Are the Benefits of Some Common Herbs?

Herb	Potential Benefits	Comments
Aloe vera (*Aloe vulgari*) (*Aloe barbadensis*)	Used topically for sunburn, wound healing, and skin irritation. Can treat constipation. Enhances immune response. Treats diabetic ulcers, asthma, and diabetes.	Antifungal, antibacterial, anti-inflammatory properties. Stimulates connective tissue formation. Not effective for asthma if taking corticosteroids.
Bilberry (*Vaccinum myrtillus*)	Acts as a potent antioxidant. Promotes retinal health. Strengthens vascular walls. Enhances circulatory systems.	May help with diabetic retinopathy or cataract formation. Its deep purple pigment contains a flavonoid compound known as anthocyanosides which are strong antioxidants to protect the eyes from free radical damage. Usual dosage: 80 mg two to four times per day
Cascara sagrada (*Rhamnus purchiana*)	Acts as an effective laxative. Helps chronic constipation.	Found in many over-the-counter laxatives.
Echinacea (*Echinacea angustifolia*) (*Echinacea purpurea*)	Potent antibacterial and antiviral. Effective for colds, flu, most infections including kidney, vaginal, tonsil, and bronchial.	Stimulates immune system. Widely used medicinal plant for various conditions. A rest period of 1–2 weeks is recommended after every 6–8 weeks of use. Usual dosage: 250 mg capsules, two times per day or 1–4 ml as a tincture.
Feverfew (*Tanacetum parthenium*)	Relieves headaches. Helps arthritis. Reduces fever. Relieves colds.	Flowers may be dried and used as an insecticide. Should not be used during pregnancy. Look for a capsule standardized to contain at least 0.2% parthenolide. Usual dosage: 100 mg capsules two or three times per day.
Garlic (*Allium sativum*)	Reduces high blood pressure. Reduces high cholesterol. Reduces high triglycerides. Prevents colds and other infections.	Antibacterial, antiviral, antifungal. May have immune-enhancing and anticancer effects.
Ginger (*Zingiber officinale*)	Treats nausea and vomiting. Helps motion sickness and digestive upset. Has anti-inflammatory properties. Supports circulation by inhibiting platelet aggregation. Useful in atherosclerosis. Prevents ulcers.	May be used as a food, plant, or medicine. Usual dosage: 250–500 mg capsules, two or three times per day.
Ginkgo biloba	Increases circulation. Acts as a powerful antioxidant. Inhibits platelet aggregation. Combats mental fatigue. Improves memory. Acts as an anti-asthmatic. Enhances blood supply to the brain. Reduces dizziness.	Derived from one of the oldest leaf-bearing trees in North America. May slow the progression of Alzheimer's disease. May reduce ringing in the ears (known as tinnitus). Perhaps the most commonly prescribed herb in all of Europe. Should not be taken at the same time as anticoagulants such as warfarin or aspirin. Usual dosage: 80 mg capsules, two or three times per day. As a tincture, 0.5 ml three times per day.

Herb	Potential Benefits	Comments
Goldenseal (*Hydrastis canadensis*)	Helps digestive disorders. Benefits morning sickness. Treats acne and eczema. Helps inflamed eyes. Treats colds and flu. Treats infectious diarrhea. Stimulates the immune system.	Has antiseptic properties which soothe and heal wounds and inflamed mucous membranes. Has antibiotic properties. Augments cancer therapies. Excessive amounts can cause gastrointestinal upset, high blood pressure, or an irregular heart rhythm. Should not be used by pregnant or lactating women. Usual dosage: 250 mg capsules two times per day.
Grape seed extract	Acts as a potent antioxidant. Protects against hardening of the arteries. Treats varicose veins. Treats retina disorders. Reduces bruising. Has anti-allergy effect. Reduces heavy menses.	An excellent source of proanthocyanidins (PCOs), a type of flavonoid. Usual dosage: 50 mg capsules, one to three per day. Improves gastrointestinal tract absorption.
Green tea (*Camellia sinensis*)	Acts as a potent antioxidant. May prevent stomach, lung, breast, prostate, pancreatic, and colon cancers.	Contains high amount of polyphenols, which can inhibit cancer-causing genes and neutralize cancer-causing chemicals. Available as both a tea or in capsule form. Catechins, which are powerful antioxidants, are the primary polyphenols found in green tea. Usual dosage: 2–4 cups of tea per day, or 100 mg capsules, two to three times per day. May protect against heart disease and stroke.
Hawthorn (*Crataegus oxycantha*)	Improves rheumatism. Treats angina. Reduces high blood pressure. Prevents atherosclerosis. Improves circulation in the legs. Improves pumping capacity of the heart. Helpful in early congestive heart failure. Potent antioxidant.	May be used for an extended period of time. High flavonoid content.
Kava Kava	Reduces stress and anxiety. Improves your mood. May help with insomnia.	Look for kava standardized to contain 30–70% kavalactones. Should not be taken by pregnant or nursing women. Usual dosage: 250 mg capsules, one to two times per day.
Milk thistle (*Silybum marianum*)	Protects and detoxifies liver. Aids regeneration of liver cells. Benefits cirrhosis of the liver.	Protects against chemical toxins and liver damage due to excess alcohol consumption. Useful in hepatitis and elevated liver enzymes. Look for standardized extract of 70% silymarin. Usual dosage: 200 mg capsules, one to three times per day.
Panax ginseng (*Korean ginseng*)	Combats mental and physical stress. Improves mental and physical performance. Helps diabetes. Combats fatigue.	Stimulates central nervous system. Lowers blood sugar. Women may experience breast tenderness at high doses. Usual dosage: 250 mg capsules, two times per day.
Pot marigold (*Calendula officinalis*)	Treats cuts, burns. Improves eczema. Reduces acne scars. Treats hemorrhoids.	Antibiotic effect fights germs, disinfects, and promotes healing.
Saw palmetto (*Serenoa repens*)	Treats enlarged prostate. (BPH). Exhibits diuretic properties.	Increases urine flow while decreasing night urination. May be more effective than Proscar for BPH. Can be more effective when combined with another herb, *Pygeum africanum*. Look for a standardized extract of 85–90% fatty acids and sterols. Usual dosage: 160 mg capsules, two per day.

Herb	Potential Benefits	Comments
Siberian ginseng (*Eleutherococcus senticosus*)	Treats exhaustion, stress, and depression. Provides a sense of rejuvenation. Stimulates central nervous system, gonads, and endocrine system, especially the pituitary and adrenals.	May benefit those with chronic fatigue syndrome. May help to lower high cholesterol levels, blood pressure, and reduce angina symptoms. Usual dosage: 100–250 mg capsules, two times per day.
St. John's wort (*Hypericum perforatum*)	Can treat mild to moderate depression. Can lift your spirits and improve your mood. Provides antiviral activity. Exhibits antibacterial properties. Assists wound healing when used topically.	May help treat herpes simplex types I and II. May treat retroviruses. Do not take if you are pregnant or breastfeeding. Look to purchase a standardized extract containing 0.3 percent hypercin and hyperforin, the active ingredients in St. John's wort. The most common antidepressant recommended in Germany. Usual dosage: 300 mg capsules, two or three times per day.
Uva Ursi	Helps treat urinary tract infections. Has a mild diuretic effect.	Urinary antiseptic and anesthetic-like effect. Not recommended during pregnancy or lactation. Do not take longer than 14 days. Usual dosage: 250–500 mg capsules, 3 times per day.
Valerian (*Valeriana officinalis*)	Helps insomnia. Alleviates anxiety. Treats menstrual cramps. Acts as a potent sedative. Acts as an antispasmodic.	Begin with a low dose, increasing dosage until effective. Do not use longer than 2 weeks. Do not take with alcohol. Usual dosage: 250–500 mg capsules, 1 hour before bedtime.

What Are Some of the Conditions That Respond to Herbal Therapy?

The following is a list of conditions that can be prevented or treated with herbs.

CONDITIONS TREATABLE WITH HERBS

Condition	Herbs
Alcoholism	Valerian, alfalfa, milk thistle (silymarin)
Atherosclerosis	Gugalipid, ginseng, hawthorn, curcumin, grape seed extract, green tea, Siberian ginseng, ginger
Antiseptic	Bay laurel, myrrh, thyme
Anxiety	Valerian, passionflower, kava kava
Arthritis	Devil's claw, boswellia, oil of evening primrose, burdock root, nettles, licorice
Asthma	Ephedra with lobelia, licorice, ginkgo biloba
Blood pressure	Garlic, hawthorn, coleus forskholii
Bronchitis	Echinacea, licorice root, chamomile, goldenseal, slippery elm
Burns	Calendula ointment, aloe vera, comfrey
Cholesterol (high)	Garlic, gugulipid, ginger
Circulation (poor)	Ginkgo biloba, garlic, cayenne, hawthorn
Colds/flu	Echinacea, astragalus, garlic, goldenseal root, licorice, yarrow
Constipation	Aloe, cascara sagrada, psyllium, dandelion, rhubarb, senna
Coughs	Licorice, wild cherry bark, thyme
Depression (mild)	St. John's wort, valerian, kava kava
Detoxification	Milk thistle (silymarin), red clover, dandelion
Diarrhea	Raspberry leaf, basil, goldenseal, carob pod powder
Digestion (poor)	Chamomile, peppermint, ginger, milk thistle, dandelion root
Expectorant	Garlic, hyssop, lobelia, licorice
Fatigue	Panax ginseng, Siberian ginseng
Fever	Echinacea, burdock, chamomile, peppermint oil

Condition	Herbs
Gall bladder	Dandelion root, chamomile, silymarin, peppermint oil
Headache	Chamomile, fennel, ginger, rose hip, valerian, willow bark
Hemorrhoids	Horse chestnut, witch hazel (topical), calendula ointment
Immune system	Echinacea, ginseng, gotu kola, astragalus, Pau D'Arco, goldenseal, garlic
Insomnia	Valerian, passionflower, hops, kava, St. John's wort, oat straw
Liver dysfunction	Milk thistle (silymarin), chelidonium, ginger, turmeric, ginseng, berberine
Memory loss	Gingko biloba, gotu kola
Menopause	Black cohosh, chasteberry, dong quai
Migraine headache	Feverfew, ginger, thyme, lavender oil
Menstrual irregularities/PMS	Dong quai, oil of evening primrose, chamomile, licorice root, chasteberry, black cohosh
Nausea	Ginger, chamomile, peppermint
Prostate enlargement (benign)	Saw palmetto, pygeum africanum, stinging nettle root
Rheumatoid arthritis	Bromelain, curcumin, ginger capsicum (topical)
Skin infections	Calendula, chamomile (topical), tea tree oil (topical)
Sore throat	Hyssop tea, lemon balm, sage gargle, slippery elm
Sunburn	Aloe vera, calendula
Stress/tension	Valerian, passionflower, kava kava, ginseng
Ulcers	Licorice, aloe juice, chamomile, comfrey, peppermint oil
Urinary tract problems	Cranberry, uva ursi
Varicose veins	Bilberry, calendula ointment, grape seed extract, bromelain, horse chestnut
Water retention	Uva ursi, dandelion leaf, saw palmetto
Yeast infections	Uva ursi, echinacea, goldenseal, cranberry, garlic

CHAPTER 19

Super Nutrients

Super nutrients play an important role in enhancing our health and improving our sense of well-being. This chapter provides a brief overview of several key therapeutic substances for achieving optimum health. These substances are generally not considered vitamins or minerals but are classified as "food components."

Alpha-Lipoic Acid

Alpha-lipoic acid is a potent antioxidant that helps neutralize the harmful effects of free radicals. It enhances the antioxidant activity of vitamins C and E as well as the enzyme glutathione. It assists the conversion of food into energy and is important in maintaining normal blood sugars. In addition, it has been effective in preventing and treating diabetic neuropathies. Alpha-lipoic acid also assists the liver in detoxification, supports the nervous system, and helps provide energy within muscles.

Bee Pollen and Propolis

Both bee pollen and propolis are produced from flowering plants and gathered by bees. They have natural antibacterial properties and help to stimulate the immune system. Many have found that these nutrients help to reduce fatigue, protect against allergies, and protect the mucous membranes from inflammation.

Blue-Green Algae

Blue-green algae is a nutrient-dense food derived from freshwater algae that is particularly high in vitamins, minerals, amino acids, protein, and chlorophyll. It has been reported to increase energy, improve mental clarity and sleep, assist assimilation and digestion, reduce stress, and strengthen the immune system.

Bovine Cartilage

Bovine cartilage helps to accelerate wound healing and to reduce inflammation. It appears to stimulate the immune system, and has been used clinically to treat conditions such as arthritis, psoriasis, and ulcerative colitis.

Chlorella

Chlorella is derived from a single-cell algae that is particularly high in chlorophyll, B vitamins, vitamin C, trace minerals, and amino acids. It is particularly high in vitamin B_{12}. It has been found to clear toxins from the bloodstream and to protect against the damaging effects of radiation.

Cod Liver Oil

Cod liver oil is high in omega-3 fatty acids, containing eicosapentaenoic acid (EPA) and docosahexaenoic acid (DHA), along with vitamins A and D. Omega-3 oil has been shown to have anti-inflammatory properties. Cod liver oil has been useful in treating dry skin and excessive buildup of earwax, and in treating children who are troubled with recurrent infections. As a result of its vitamin A and vitamin D content, excessive doses of cod liver oil can be toxic.

Creatine

Creatine is a nutritional supplement frequently used to support athletic performance, commonly for short-duration, high-intensity workouts. Creatine supplements increase the intracellular levels of creatine phosphate, a compound used to make ATP and the body's main source of energy during exercise. It appears that creatine monohydrate can increase the level of creatine in your muscle stores so that you can produce more ATP. Creatine monohydrate has been particularly helpful for those involved in short sprint performances, power lifting, and other forms of high-intensity training. Red meat is one of the main dietary sources of creatine. However, supplements are available that are free of fat and cholesterol. As a dietary supplement, I usually recommend taking up to 20 grams per day for five to seven days and then continuing a maintenance dose of 5–10 grams daily for a short period of time.

DHA (Docosahexaenoic acid)

DHA, an omega-3 fatty acid typically derived from fish oil concentrates or flaxseed oil, is important in nourishing both the brain and the retina. It is also helpful in improving sight in infants and learning capacity. DHA occurs naturally in breast milk and infants who are exclusively fed with formulas may be deficient. This may account for the reason that breast-fed babies generally develop better visual acuity at an earlier age than formula-fed infants. I have found that DHA can help cognitive performance in children and adults and has been useful in the treatment of attention deficit disorder, autism, and Down syndrome.

DMG (Dimethylglycine)

DMG is also known as pangamic acid or vitamin B_{15}. Clinically, it has been used to improve oxygenation, mental acuity, and immune function, and to maintain energy levels. DMG is helpful in controlling epileptic seizures and may be useful in the treatment of autism. Some athletes report that it improves their endurance.

Evening Primrose Oil

Evening primrose oil is particularly high in gamma-linoleic acid (GLA), an omega-6 fatty acid. It has been useful in treating premenstrual tension and relieving symptoms of allergies, arthritis, eczema, and autoimmune disorders. Recently, it has been shown to be of benefit to children who have been diagnosed with attention deficit disorder, hyperactivity, and dyslexia. It may also be effective in treating fibrocystic breast disease, premenstrual tension, and dysmenorrhea (painful menstrual periods). Other sources of GLA include borage oil and black currant oil.

Fish Oils

Fish oils are particularly high in omega-3 fatty acids. These oils contain both EPA (eicosapentaneoic acid) and DHA (docosahexaenoic acid). Fish oils function as anti-inflammatories and have been useful in reducing symptoms of arthritis, lowering cholesterol and triglyceride levels, reducing platelet stickiness, and reducing the symptoms of ulcerative colitis. In some cases, fish oils have been reported to reduce the symptoms associated with organ rejection after transplant and may prevent the closing up of the coronary arteries after an angioplasty. Omega-3 fatty acids are primarily found in cold-water fish such as salmon, cod, tuna, herring, and mackerel.

Flaxseed Oil

Flaxseed oil is a good source of omega-3 fatty acids and, in particular, alpha-linolenic acid. The seeds are particularly high in fiber and are helpful in treating constipation, irritable bowel syndrome, and digestive troubles such as inflammatory bowel disease and spastic colon. Flaxseed oil helps promote strong bones and healthy skin, and has been used to treat a variety of skin conditions, including eczema and psoriasis. Make sure you store flaxseed oil in the refrigerator and never use it in cooking.

FOS (Fructo-Oligosaccharides)

FOS is a probiotic that enhances the capabilities of the digestive tract. It helps maintain a healthy intestinal environment and promotes the growth of the naturally occurring friendly bacteria lactobacillus acidophilus and bifidus.

Glucosamine Sulfate and Chondroitin Sulfate

Both glucosamine sulfate and chondroitin sulfate are vital components of healthy connective tissue and have been used to treat rheumatoid arthritis and osteoarthritis. They support healthy joints and may stimulate the production of new cartilage.

Grape Seed Extract

Grape seed extract is a potent source of proanthocyanidins, a naturally occurring substance with powerful antioxidant properties. It strengthens capillaries and connective tissue, acts as an antifungal, and also functions as an anti-inflammatory.

"Green Drinks"

"Green drinks" are a combination of various plant substances that detoxify and cleanse the bloodstream. They are generally rich in chlorophyll, vitamins, minerals, and enzymes. Many contain a variety of grasses such as alfalfa, barley, or wheat grass. In addition, they may contain spirulina, kelp, blue-green algae, chlorella, and a variety of other important nutrients. It has been reported that these drinks help increase vitality and energy, enhance the immune response, and promote a sense of well-being.

Green Tea

Green tea contains numerous antioxidant compounds known as polyphenols. Polyphenols, which are actually a type of flavonoid, protect the body against the harmful effects of free radicals. Green tea has been reported to reduce the risk of cardiovascular disease, lower cholesterol levels, and protect against cancer. The beneficial effects of green tea have been attributed to the high content of catechin, a specific polyphenol with strong antioxidant potential.

Horse Chestnut Extract

Horse chestnut extract helps to support healthy circulation of the legs and has been used to treat varicose veins and chronic venous insufficiency. It supports the overall health of the veins and may improve blood flow, reduce edema and leg pain, as well as combat free radical damage. You may also find that horse chestnut can help to get rid of spider veins. Escin, the active ingredient in horse chestnut extract, is responsible for promoting venous health. I generally recommend 250–500 mg of horse chestnut extract per day for at least three months for varicose veins.

5-Hydroxy L-tryptophan

5-hydroxy L-tryptophan (5-HTP) is a metabolite from tryptophan, an essential amino acid. 5-HTP is metabolized into serotonin, an important neurotransmitter involved in the regulation of numerous brain activities including emotional well-being, appetite, sleep patterns, and depression. I have found that 5-HTP can help to reduce insomnia and to encourage a good night's sleep. In doses of 100–300 mg per day, it can help to reduce depression and elevate your mood. It is also metabolized into melatonin, a hormone that encourages sound sleep and reduces insomnia.

Ipriflavone

Ipriflavone is a synthetically derived isoflavone, which may be helpful in preventing osteoporosis. Ipriflavone not only is capable of inhibiting the breakdown of existing bone, but also can help to increase new bone formation in postmenopausal women. I generally recommend 200 mg of ipriflavone three times per day, and it can be used in conjunction with calcium, estrogen, and other bone-enhancing therapies.

Lactobacillus acidophilus and bifidus

Both *lactobacillus acidophilus* and *bifidus* are normal constituents of healthy intestinal flora. They help to synthesize B vitamins in the intestinal tract and are valuable in assisting the digestive process. They are known as "friendly" bacteria and are frequently destroyed when taking antibiotics. Lactobacillus promotes the proper digestion of foods; reduces intestinal gas, bloating, and constipation; and improves overall bowel function. Lactobacilli have also been used to prevent and treat chronic vaginal yeast infections and urinary tract infections.

Lecithin

Lecithin is a natural constituent of the fatty membranes of all cells. It is particularly high in the B vitamins choline and inositol. Lecithin has been used to prevent cardiovascular disease, to improve brain function, and to protect the liver against the ill effects of alcoholism. It helps to emulsify fats and may help to reduce cholesterol and triglyceride levels.

Maitake Mushrooms (*Grifola frondosa*)

Maitake mushrooms have been used by the Chinese and Japanese cultures for centuries. Their powerful effect has been attributed to their high concentrations of a polysaccharide called Beta-1, 6-Glucan, which has been shown to stimulate the immune system. In laboratory studies, Maitake mushroom extracts have been shown to inhibit cancerous tumor growth and to enhance the activity of key immune cells known as T-helper cells. These mushrooms have also been found to be useful in the treatment of chronic fatigue syndrome, diabetes, HIV infections, high blood pressure, allergies, obesity, constipation, and chronic hepatitis. The protein-bound extract of maitake mushroom known as D-fraction is the most immune-enhancing portion of the mushroom.

MSM (Methyl-Sulfonyl-Methane or Dimethyl Sulfone)

MSM is a naturally occurring compound that contains organic sulfur, an important component of healthy skin, connective tissue, and the immune system. Sulfur plays a significant role in the formation of collagen and keratin including joints, hair, skin, and nails. Although naturally occurring MSM can be found in natural and processed foods, any processing including heating or frying can reduce the biological activity of MSM. Clinically, MSM has been important in arthritic conditions and may improve overall joint mobility. I have also used it in allergic conditions, primarily for pollen sensitivity. It may also have an immune-enhancing effect and reduce the need for steroids or antibiotics. Doses from 1,000 to 3,000 mg per day can provide help for pain, stiffness, inflammation, and swelling of the joints.

NADH

NADH (*nicotinamide adenine dinucleotide*) is a substance that is naturally used within the Krebs cycle, one of the main biochemical pathways that helps you convert fat and sugar into energy. NADH is showing promising results in improving function in people with Alzheimer's disease, Parkinson's disease, and chronic fatigue.

Octacosanol

Octacosanol is derived from wheat germ oil concentrate and increases the utilization of oxygen during heavy exercise. It may improve muscle recovery, reduce pain after exercise, and increase physical endurance.

Olive Leaf Extract

Olive leaf extract is thought to be a strong immune system booster. It has been found to alleviate sore throats, sinus infections, and has antiviral, antibacterial, and antifungal properties. The beneficial properties are thought to be due to the compound oleuropein and its active ingredient, oleanolic acid. I have found that olive leaf extract may be more effective than antibiotics with fewer side effects. I generally recommend 250–500 mg per day to help prevent or combat infections.

Phosphatidylserine (PS)

The human brain contains high concentrations of the nutrient phosphatidylserine (PS). It is commonly called a "brain nutrient" since it may improve cognitive function, improve mood, fight depression, and boost memory. It has been found to improve the quality of life in Alzheimer's patients and to revitalize brain and neurologic function. It is quite safe and well tolerated. I usually recommend 100 mg three times per day.

Pycnogenol®

Pycnogenol® is a registered trademark name referring specifically to the extract from the bark of the French maritime pine tree. It is high in proanthocyanidins (PCOs), which are naturally occurring food and botanical substances that are high in the antioxidants known as flavonols. Pycnogenol has been reported to strengthen blood vessels, improve blood circulation, assist with varicose veins, protect against bruising, improve joint flexibility, and help promote healing.

Quercetin

Quercetin is a bioflavonoid with anti-inflammatory properties. It has been used to treat allergic conditions such as itchy watery eyes or nasal congestion and to help reduce the symptoms of asthma. It may also be valuable in lowering the risk of developing cataracts and viruses. Quercetin may protect you from the adverse effects of LDL cholesterol. It is found in foods such as broccoli, apples, tomatoes, green peppers, and onions.

Red Yeast Rice

The extract of red yeast fermented on rice has been a traditional Chinese remedy that has been used for more than 1,000 years for circulatory health. It may help to lower the total cholesterol, LDL or "bad" cholesterol, and raise the HDL or "good" cholesterol. Marketed as cholestin, this substance contains naturally occurring HMG-CoA reductase inhibitors which assist the metabolism of cholesterol. Although red yeast rice should not be used during pregnancy or lactation, it is generally well tolerated. However, a small percentage have complained of mild gastrointestinal problems or headaches. Overall, I have found that red yeast rice can be successfully used as an alternative for commonly prescribed cholesterol-lowering drugs.

Resveratrol

Resveratrol, a compound found in the skin of red grapes and in red wine, provides potent antioxidant properties to these foods. In fact, resveratrol may be responsible for part of the cholesterol-lowering effect attributed to red wine. Resveratrol has a cardioprotective effect by inhibiting platelet aggregation. It also modulates prostaglandin synthesis and inhibits inflammatory pathways. Resveratrol may also have an anticancer effect by activating p53, a protein that has been linked to protection against cancer. It can be used in conjunction with other antioxidants to help protect against free radical damage.

SAMe

SAMe, or S-adenosyl-methionine, a compound produced in the body from methionine and ATP, has been used both to improve joint health as well as mood. Vitamin B_{12} and folic acid also serve as cofactors in the production of SAMe. I have found it to be successful in the treatment of depression, often more effective than conventional antidepressants. SAMe has also been useful to treat osteoarthritis and may be more effective than taking nonsteroidal anti-inflammatory drugs. You should not put SAMe in the refrigerator since it can add moisture and therefore accelerate oxidation of the supplement. For mild to moderate depression or osteoarthritis, I recommend taking 200–800 mg of SAMe per day. Doses up to 1,600 mg per day may be necessary for major depression. At higher doses, you might find that SAMe can cause mild headaches or occasional loose bowels. Overall, however, it appears to be a very safe and effective supplement.

Shark Cartilage

Shark cartilage contains biologically active proteins that have been reported to inhibit the growth of tumors. It accomplishes this by suppressing the development of new blood vessels, thereby depriving the tumor of oxygen and nutrients, components necessary for tumor growth. Shark cartilage may also be useful in the treatment of arthritis, psoriasis, and colitis. It also contains substances that stimulate the immune system.

Shiitake and Reishi Mushrooms

Both shiitake (*Lentinus edodes*) and reishi mushrooms (*Ganoderma lucidum*) are widely used in the Far East. They have been associated with improved vitality and enhanced immune function. They may help to reduce the risk of heart disease and high blood pressure, lower blood cholesterol, reduce fatigue, and lower susceptibility to viral infections. Owing to their antitumor properties, these mushrooms may be useful in treating cancers.

Tocotrienols

Tocotrienols, which are quite rich in rice bran oil, are compounds that are structurally related to vitamin E but have distinct functions of their own. Tocotrienols are most well known for their cardiovascular support by helping to lower blood cholesterol levels. They do this by modulating the main enzyme involved in cholesterol synthesis, HMG-CoA reductase activity. I have found this substance to have a positive effect on lowering cholesterol levels, and it may be even more effective than some of the pharmaceutical agents commonly used to lower cholesterol. Overall, tocotrienols and vitamin E work well together to support cardiovascular health and to provide antioxidant protection.

CHAPTER 20

Two Remarkable Therapies: Homeopathy and Chelation Therapy

> *The highest ideal of cure is the speedy, gentle and enduring restoration of health by the most trustworthy and least harmful way.*
>
> —Samuel Hahnemann (1755–1844),
> founder of homeopathy

Two healing techniques that are gaining increased recognition are homeopathy, which is over 200 years old, and chelation therapy, a more recent non-surgical treatment. Both work slowly—but very differently—and both can assist in healing a variety of conditions.

What Is Homeopathy?

Homeopathic medicine was developed by the well-respected German physician and chemist Dr. Samuel Hahnemann. At the turn of the century, homeopathy was widely accepted and one out of every five doctors prescribed homeopathic remedies on a regular basis. Homeopathy hit a twenty-year lull between 1950 and 1970. However, since the 1970s, the need for noninvasive, less costly medicines and cures were the major catalysts that reignited the resurgence of homeopathic medicine. The use of homeopathic remedies in the United States is now growing rapidly.

Homeopathy is a unique system of medicine that is based on the Laws of Similars. That is, the same substance that in large doses causes an illness can cure the same illness if given in small or nearly infinitesimal amounts. For example, if you are troubled with poison ivy, taking a homeopathic preparation of Rhus Toxicodendron (from the poison ivy plant) may help to reduce your symptoms.

Homeopathic medications are generally referred to as "remedies." They are commonly prepared from plants, herbs, flowers, minerals, viruses, bacteria, or animal products and are thought to stimulate your body's own natural defenses. There are hundreds of different homeopathic remedies available at a variety of different dosages or strengths. Selecting the correct remedy is the task of a skilled homeopath. However, these remedies are so safe that if the improper remedy is selected, it would have virtually no adverse effect on your body. When prescribed correctly, they can act quite rapidly and be curative, simulating your body's defenses rather than simply suppressing symptoms.

Homeopathic remedies are generally prepared by diluting different plant products thousands of times. In addition, they are succussed (repeatedly shaken and pounded on a hard surface) at the same time. Succussing is thought to instill energy into the homeopathic remedy. Oddly enough, the more diluted and succussed a remedy is, the more potent it becomes. This is in direct contrast to Western medications where stronger doses are more potent and have a greater impact on your body.

Can Anyone Use Homeopathic Medicine?

Virtually anyone can take homeopathic remedies. They have been used effectively in treating infants, children, adults, and senior citizens. Common problems that may be amenable to homeopathic treatments include a wide variety of acute and chronic problems such as chronic infections, allergies, gynecologic complaints, premenstrual tension, headaches, skin problems, gastrointestinal complaints, and fever.

There are actually two major types of prescribing by a skilled homeopath. For more chronic, ongoing problems, a "constitutional remedy" may be recommended. This type of remedy takes into account the uniqueness of the individual. For example, your emotions, feelings, likes and dislikes, desires and fears may be factors in deciding what remedy may be best for you. On the other hand, acute prescribing of a homeopathic remedy is usually done for more acute symptoms such as a sudden infection; a high fever; a migraine headache; a cut, scrape, or burn; or a cough.

Taking Homeopathic Remedies

Interestingly, a single remedy may be used to treat a variety of different health conditions. When taking a homeopathic history, all symptoms are taken into account since they can all have an impact on the body's effort to heal itself. Remedies are usually taken in the form of small pellets, tinctures, or in some cases, are even applied topically. As a general rule, it is recommended that you do not touch the pellets with your hands. The liquids are placed under the tongue. It is best not to have any water or food for at least 30 minutes before or after taking the remedy. You should also avoid drinking coffee, mint, or spicy foods while taking homeopathic remedies. Once you feel the desired effect, i.e., your cough has gone away or you are no longer nauseous, you should stop taking the medication. On occasion, you may feel worse when you initially take your remedy. This is called an aggravation and is thought to be a normal sign that your body's healing defenses are being activated.

Although homeopathy has been in existence for more than 200 years, it still remains a controversial treatment. However, I have found it to be extremely useful in treating my patients for some of the most common ailments that I see. This can include the treatment of sinus infections, congestion, headaches, menopausal symptoms, irregular menstrual periods, PMS, headaches, and even arthritic pains. Although some authorities feel that homeopathic remedies should only be taken alone and not combined with any other treatment, I have found that these therapies work quite well in conjunction with other herbal treatments and nutritional supplements. You can readily find homeopathic remedies in your local health food store or in many pharmacies.

You can usually find a well-qualified homeopath through a recommendation from your local health food store or by contacting the associations which are listed in Appendix III.

What Is Chelation Therapy?

Chelation therapy involves the administration of an intravenous solution that is given in a doctor's office over three to four hours on a regular basis. Many patients require between twenty and thirty treatments before noticing favorable results. Chelation therapy utilizes a mixture of vitamins, minerals, and a synthetically derived amino acid known as EDTA (ethylene-diaminetetraacetic acid). This solution helps to reduce free radical formation and to remove excess intra-arterial calcium, excess iron, lead, copper, and other heavy metals. To be most effective, chelation therapy must be combined with proper diet, exercise, stress reduction, and an individualized oral vitamin and mineral program. It is also imperative that smoking be completely eliminated for this therapy to be effective.

In contrast to bypass surgery, which treats only a specific segment of an artery, chelation therapy treats all the arteries of the body simultaneously. This leads to improved circulation to the brain, heart, legs, and all organs of the body. I have treated hundreds of patients who, after being told they needed bypass surgery by their cardiologist or cardiac surgeon, have opted instead to have chelation therapy. Many of these patients have had complete resolution of their chest pain, leg pain, shortness of breath, and a variety of other symptoms. In fact, one of the major benefits that I have noted is a reduction in medications for patients receiving chelation therapy.

While EDTA chelation therapy has been FDA approved for lead toxicity, its efficacy for treating other disorders is controversial. It is crucial that EDTA be administered and monitored by highly trained medical personnel under the care of a qualified physician.

What Are the Benefits of Chelation Therapy?

Although the biochemical mechanisms may not be fully understood, chelation therapy appears to:

- Improve circulation.
- Reduce the stickiness of platelets.
- Reduce the risk of blood clots or thrombosis.
- Quench free radical damage.
- Remove toxic metals such as lead and cadmium from the body.
- Remove excess iron and copper, elements implicated in free radical damage.
- Alleviate chest pain (angina pectoris).
- Relieve pain and cramps in the legs.
- Reduce generalized fatigue.
- Enhance memory.

SOME OF THE MOST COMMON AILMENTS SUCCESSFULLY TREATED INCLUDE:

- Lead poisoning.
- Coronary artery disease.
- Arteriosclerosis.
- High blood pressure.
- High cholesterol.
- Peripheral vascular disease.
- Carotid artery disease.
- Angina pectoris.

Is There Scientific Evidence Supporting Chelation Therapy?

The scientific evidence in support of chelation therapy is mounting. It has been estimated that more than 800,000 people have undergone this therapy, with approximately 80 percent experiencing clinical benefits. There are at least forty studies highlighting the benefits of chelation therapy, although many of these have been criticized by opponents of chelation therapy since most are not double-blinded studies. The following summaries may give you insight into the efficacy of chelation therapy.

- A double-blind study of chelation therapy involving ten patients with peripheral vascular disease was reported in the *Journal of the National Medical Association*. Five patients received chelation therapy and the other half had a placebo. After ten treatments, the patients receiving chelation therapy showed dramatic improvement. They were able to walk farther and there was improved circulation in the extremities. Because of these results, the study was changed to single-blind. For the next ten treatments, both groups were given chelation therapy. The study stated that the subjects that originally received placebo, but later received chelation therapy, showed similar improvement to those patients who were in the original chelation group.

- Information reported in *Medical Hypothesis* looked at 2,870 patients and stated that 93.5 percent of heart patients showed a marked improvement after receiving chelation therapy. The same report stated that 98.5 percent of people with circulatory problems in the legs showed marked improvement, as did 54 percent of people with brain disorders.

- An article in the *Journal for the Advancement of Medicine* reported that of 65 Swedish patients who received chelation therapy while on a waiting list for bypass surgery, 58 were able to cancel their surgery. The same article reported that of 27 patients who received chelation therapy while on a waiting list for surgical amputations, 24 were able to cancel their surgery.

- In a meta-analysis where 41 different studies using EDTA chelation therapy for vascular disease were analyzed, 87 percent of over 22,000 patients had measurable improvement after chelation therapy treatments.

CHAPTER 21

Treating Common Illnesses Naturally

After practicing medicine for twenty years, I can proudly say that most medical conditions seen in a family practice setting can be effectively treated without the use of prescription medications. Even to this day, I am still in awe of the power of natural healing therapies. Patients who are motivated to eat nutrient-dense, antioxidant-rich, wholesome foods and exercise on a regular basis are certainly those who respond better to natural therapies. Effectively handling stress and practicing some form of mind-body exercises such as yoga or meditation are also essential aspects of feeling healthy. In addition, I have found that the judicious use of appropriate vitamins, minerals, herbal therapies, and homeopathics are an integral part in helping to prevent or reverse some of the most common ailments affecting the public today. These natural healing techniques can also help to slow the aging process and increase the number of quality years that you strive for.

This chapter will discuss up-to-date, cutting-edge, natural therapies for some of the most common maladies or health problems that you may encounter. Hopefully, by applying the principles discussed in this book, most of these health complaints can be minimized or, better yet, completely avoided.

I have provided two lists of the nutritional supplements that I have found most important in combating each health concern, with my first choice labeled "Highly Recommended." If you find that these nutrients are not as efficacious as you would like, then consider trying my suggestions labeled "Often Recommended." These, too, have shown great promise in many cases.

Keep in mind that these are general guidelines based on my twenty years of experience in successfully treating more than 10,000 patients at the Magaziner Center for Wellness and Anti-Aging Medicine in Cherry Hill, New Jersey, and the latest advances in medical and nutritional research. You may be able to find supplements that contain many of my recommended nutrients in one pill rather than having to take each nutrient separately. In addition, even if a multiple vitamin with minerals was not listed as a suggestion for each health problem, I recommend that virtually everyone take at least a multivitamin on a regular basis.

Lastly, the doses that I have recommended may need to be adjusted depending on your weight, metabolism, age, stress level, family history, and other factors since your biochemical needs and genetics are unique. For example, women who are or could become pregnant should not take more than 10,000 IU of vitamin A per day.

I have used most of the vitamins, minerals, herbs, and other nutrients I have suggested to combat the medical conditions discussed in this chapter. However, I will also define and emphasize the importance of some cutting-edge products that you may not be aware of.

Acne

Acne, the most common of all skin disorders, is characterized by inflammation, redness, blackheads (comedones), and whiteheads (pustules). Acne frequently affects the face, neck, shoulders, or back in teenagers and young adults. This condition is frequently triggered when the hormone testosterone is secreted at puberty. Acne can also be triggered if the skin pores become blocked and the bacteria *Propionibacterium acnes* flourish and release enzymes that promote inflammation. Although acne affects both males and females, males are more prone to the condition.

At times, because food allergies may exacerbate your acne, it is important to identify what foods you are allergic to. In addition, I strongly recommend that you eliminate all refined sugar and trans-fatty acids from your diet. The following are some of the nutrients which I have found to be helpful:

Highly Recommended:

Zinc: 30–50 mg per day

Vitamin A: 25,000–50,000 IU per day (Higher doses should be monitored, and if you are pregnant, your dose should not exceed 10,000 IU.)

Selenium: 200-400 mcg per day

Vitamin E: 400 IU per day

Often Recommended:

Vitamin B_6: 50 mg per day

Azelaic acid (20% topical preparation): Apply twice a day

Pantothenic acid: 1,000 mg three times per day

Tea tree oil: Apply topically twice a day

Health Tip: Azelaic Acid

Azelaic acid is a compound that has antibacterial effects for the skin and can be used to treat acne problems. It is available both by prescription or from Cardiovascular Research. (See Resource Guide.)

Health Tip: Tea Tree Oil

Tea tree oil is derived from the leaves of a tall evergreen tree that grows in Australia and Asia. The oil helps kill fungus and bacteria, and weak dilutions at 5–15 percent can be used topically for the treatment of acne. Keep tea tree oil away from your eyes.

Allergies

Over thirty-five million Americans suffer from allergies. Allergies involve an inappropriate response to the inhalation or ingestion of or contact with a specific substance, which provokes the immune system to defend itself. The allergenic substance is frequently not harmful or troublesome to a nonallergic individual. An allergy sufferer might experience nasal congestion, wheezing, itchy eyes, coughing, headaches, hives or skin rashes, generalized complaints of fatigue, muscle aches and pains, digestive difficulties, headaches, or an inability to concentrate.

Almost any substance can cause an allergic response in a susceptible individual. However, the most common inhalant allergies include grass, trees or weed pollen, dust, house dust mites, molds, animal dander, and chemical odors such as cigarette smoke and perfume. Food can also be a common trigger of allergic responses. Milk, wheat, soy, peanuts, chocolate, eggs, corn, shellfish, strawberries, and yeast are just a few of the foods that seem particularly troublesome. An increasing number of individuals are having adverse reactions to cleaning agents, paints, solvents, construction material, insecticides, and pesticides.

In order to reduce your allergy symptoms, it is important that your immune system function at peak levels. Vitamin C with bioflavonoids, if taken in appropriate doses, can have a powerful antihistamine-like effect. The bioflavonoid quercitin appears particularly important in enhancing the immune response against allergies. Calcium, magnesium, pantothenic acid, zinc, and essential fatty acids such as flaxseed, borage, and primrose oil can also be effective in supporting the immune system and warding off allergies. B-complex vitamins and antioxidants will also enhance immune response. Vitamin E, Coenzyme Q_{10}, and acidophilus with bifidus are especially effective for upper respiratory allergy symptoms and for recurrent infections. The herbs echinacea, goldenseal, and stinging nettle may also be effective to help strengthen the immune system and reduce your need for medications.

Try to remove all allergenic substances from the house or office and use an air purifier and less chemically contaminated cleaning agents. Read food labels and avoid food additives such as monosodium glutamate (MSG) and artificial colorings such as yellow dye No. 5, both of which have been linked to allergies. Some people have found that they need to rotate their food in order to reduce their food sensitivities.

If you are suffering from allergies, the following substances may be beneficial:

Highly Recommended:

Vitamin C: 1,000 mg three times per day
Quercetin: 500 mg three times per day
Grape seed extract: 100 mg two times per day
Bioflavonoids: 500 mg three times per day

Bromelain: 250 mg two times per day
N-acetylcysteine (NAC): 600 mg two times per day
MSM: 1,000 mg three times per day
Stinging nettle: 120 mg two times per day

Health Tip: N-acetylcysteine (NAC)

NAC is an altered form of the amino acid cysteine that helps to break up mucus. Furthermore, it aids your body in synthesizing glutathione, a potent antioxidant. NAC helps to protect the liver from the effects of toxic chemicals and can protect you from acetaminophen toxicity. I have found it helpful for people suffering from excessive mucus formation and allergies.

Often Recommended:

Zinc: 30 mg per day

Vitamin E: 400 IU per day

Vitamin B complex: 50 mg per day

Coenzyme Q_{10}: 50 mg per day

Pantothenic acid: 500 mg two times per day

Flaxseed oil: 1 tablespoon per day

Evening primrose oil: 1,300 mg two times
  per day

Alzheimer's Disease

Alzheimer's disease is a degenerative brain disorder that generally affects older persons. Symptoms can include a loss of memory, difficulty learning new information, loss of interest in hobbies or everyday activities, or trouble recalling names and appointments. The disease can then progress slowly to the point where a person can be more debilitated and have difficulty getting dressed, losing interest in personal appearance, and neglecting hygiene.

There are probably several causes that contribute to Alzheimer's disease. Genetics may play a role, as specific genes have recently been identified that can increase your risk. Accelerated oxidative damage within the brain also seems to play a central role in the development of Alzheimer's disease. Continuous exposure to aluminum is another possible factor in the development of Alzheimer's disease and, therefore, should be avoided, especially since some common medications, like those used for gastrointestinal upset, contain aluminum. There is also preliminary evidence that excessive mercury accumulation can contribute to Alzheimer's. Several nutrients that may be of benefit include the following:

Highly Recommended:

Antioxidant complex: Two times per day

Ginkgo biloba: 80 mg three times per day

Vitamin B complex: 50 mg per day

Vitamin E: 400 IU per day

Acetyl-L-Carnitine: 500 mg three times
  per day

Vitamin B_{12}: 1,000 mcg two times per day

Coenzyme Q_{10}: 100 mg two times per day

Phosphatidylserine: 100 mg three times
  per day

Health Tip: Phosphatidylserine

Phosphatidylserine, a phospholipid in high concentrations in the brain, has been found to be particularly effective in improving the quality of life and enhancing memory, cognitive function, and other neurologic properties in people with Alzheimer's disease.

Health Tip: Acetyl-L-Carnitine

Acetyl-L-Carnitine is a molecule composed of acetic acid and carnitine that are bound together. Although the substance is naturally produced in the brain, supplements may be helpful in treating the early stages of Alzheimer's disease and impaired memory.

Often Recommended:

Thiamine (vitamin B_1): 3,000–8,000 mg per day

Flaxseed oil: 1 tablespoon per day

DHA: 500 mg per day

Lecithin granules: 1 tablespoon per day

NADH: 2.5 mg two or three times per day

Estrogen: By prescription from your doctor

DHEA: Under your doctor's supervision

Health Tip: DHA (docosahexaenoic acid)

DHA is an essential fatty acid high in omega-3 fats that helps to nourish the brain and retina and has been associated with improvement in cognitive function.

Health Tip: NADH (or nicotinamide adenine dinucleotide)

NADH fuels the Krebs cycle, one of the major biochemical cycles, which helps to burn fat and sugar to be converted into energy. NADH is also a coenzyme that enhances cellular energy to improve brain and neurologic function. It is a potent antioxidant and has been successfully used for Alzheimer's disease, Parkinson's disease, and chronic fatigue syndrome. NADH seems to improve alertness, concentration, emotion, and mood.

Health Tip: DHEA (Dehydroepiandrosterone)

DHEA is a naturally occurring steroid hormone produced by the adrenal gland. As it is converted into estrogen and testosterone, normal body levels of DHEA decline with the age-related decline in these two hormones. DHEA may improve energy, reduce risk of heart disease, enhance insulin utilization, reduce risk of osteoporosis, and enhance your immune response. However, since this is a hormone, it should be used only under the supervision of a health-care professional. Some women have found that taking DHEA can stimulate facial hair growth or cause facial acne.

Angina Pectoris

Angina pectoris is typically characterized by chest pain, which can also be accompanied by chest tightness or a squeezing sensation. It is usually due to insufficient oxygen being carried to the heart muscle as a result of poor blood supply from plaque buildup. Physical exertion or stress can worsen angina, so care here is a must.

In reducing angina symptoms, it is also important to eliminate cigarette smoking and to maintain your ideal body weight. It's also important to avoid eating refined carbohydrates and simple sugars.

In this regard, you may want to consider a very low-fat diet that is primarily based on plant foods such as fruit, vegetables, whole grains, beans, legumes, pasta, tofu, and other soy products. I have also found that intravenous chelation therapy can also provide an effective treatment in reducing symptoms of angina pectoris. Some of the most important nutritional supplements include:

Highly Recommended:

Magnesium citrate or aspartate: 300–400 mg twice per day

Coenzyme Q_{10}: 60–300 mg per day

Vitamin E: 400 IU twice per day

Acetyl-L-Carnitine: 500 mg three times per day

Arginine: 1,000 mg three times per day

Lysine: 500 mg three times per day

Bromelain: 500 mg three times per day

Hawthorn: 240–480 mg per day

Health Tip: Bromelain

Bromelain is an enzyme derived from pineapple and has anti-inflammatory effects. It may help to prevent the progression of the inflammatory pathways that are associated with cardiovascular disease. Bromelain can also prevent platelet stickiness, thereby reducing the risk of thrombus or blood clots.

Often Recommended:

Garlic: 1,000 mg twice per day

Flaxseed oil: 1 tablespoon twice per day

Vitamin C: 500 mg twice per day

Pantethine: 300 mg twice per day

Anxiety

Anxiety is often characterized by tightness in the chest, heart palpitations, hyperventilation, shakiness, or simply an unpleasant feeling of uneasiness or fear. Fear can also trigger headaches, muscle spasms, excessive sweating, dry mouth, or loose bowels. Reducing sugar, caffeine, alcohol, and food intolerances can greatly reduce your symptoms. Some of the most useful nutrients include the following:

Highly Recommended:

Vitamin B complex: 50 mg per day
Niacinamide: 500 mg three times per day
Calcium citrate: 500 mg one or two times per day

Magnesium: 400 mg one or two times per day
5-HTP: 100 mg three times per day
Kava: 100 mg three times per day

Often Recommended:

Vitamin B_{12}: 1,000 mcg two times per day
Inositol: 1,000 mg three times per day
GABA: 500 mg one or two times per day

St. John's wort: 300 mg two or three times per day

Health Tip: GABA

GABA (gamma-aminobutyric acid) is both an amino acid and a neurotransmitter, a chemical that sends messages from one cell to another. GABA can be used as a natural tranquilizer and can be effective for anxiety, depression, and seizure disorders.

Arthritis

Arthritis is characterized by inflammation and pain in one or more joints, frequently accompanied by deterioration of the joint cartilage. Deterioration causes the bones to rub together, thereby causing varying degrees of pain. Arthritis sufferers often complain of stiffness, pain, swelling, tenderness, reduced range of motion, or deformities of the joints.

There are various forms of arthritis. Rheumatoid arthritis is characterized by an autoimmune reaction whereby immune complexes are formed that lead to joint deterioration and destruction. This condition is found predominantly in women and usually begins before age forty. Osteoarthritis, on the other hand, begins during later stages of life and is also referred to as "wear and tear arthritis," or degenerative joint disease. The surfaces of the cartilage, which form the buffer between two bones, begin to wear away, resulting in friction and subsequent pain. Osteoarthritis can be diagnosed with the help of an x-ray and, like rheumatoid arthritis, occurs more frequently in women than men.

Both forms of arthritis may be influenced by diet. Symptoms can be reduced by elminating food allergens and improving the quality of the food. Reducing the amount of saturated fat, especially dairy products and red meat, may also be helpful. Many people with arthritis are sensitive to solanine, a substance found in nightshade vegetables. Two to three months of avoiding nightshade vegetables such as peppers, eggplant, tomatoes, and white potatoes has offered relief for many sufferers.

Dietary supplements may be helpful for reducing joint discomfort, stiffness, and pain, and reducing medication requirements. At times, nutritional supplements may even restore joint integrity. I've obtained impressive results using a good-quality multivitamin with minerals and additional vitamins C and E, along with the combination of both glucosamine sulfate and chondroitin sulfate. These supplements seem to restore normal integrity to the joints and, in particular, the cartilage. The essential fatty acids found in evening primrose oil and borage oil also have a profound anti-inflammatory effect. Trace minerals such as boron, zinc, manganese, and magnesium have proven to be beneficial. Pantothenic acid, vitamin B_6, and niacinamide are also useful in reducing the symptoms of osteoarthritis.

If you suffer from arthritis, the following supplements may be beneficial:

Highly Recommended:

Glucosamine sulfate: 500 mg three times per day

Vitamin E: 400 IU per day

Vitamin C: 1,000 mg two times per day

Pantothenic acid: 100 mg two times per day

Boron: 3 mg per day

Niacinamide: 250–500 mg three times per day

Omega-3 oils (EPA/DHA): 1,000–2,000 mg three times per day

Evening primrose oil: 1,300 mg two times per day

Bromelain: 500 mg per day

Vitamin B_6: 50 mg two times per day

MSM: 1,000 mg three times per day

Multiple vitamin with trace minerals

Antioxidant supplement

Often Recommended:

Borage oil capsules: 250 mg three times per day

Ginger: 500 mg two times per day

Boswellia: 400 mg three times per day

SAMe: 200 mg two times per day

Chondroitin sulfate: 400 mg three times per day

Sea cucumber: 1,000 mg two times per day

Curcumin: 250 mg two times per day

Health Tip: Sea Cucumber

Sea cucumber is a relative of the starfish that is typically found off the coast of Australia. Sea cucumber supplements can significantly reduce arthritic pain, joint aches, and stiffness.

Asthma

Asthma is characterized by wheezing, shortness of breath, and excessive mucus formation that occurs when the lungs become inflamed. Environmental irritants such as cigarette smoke, perfume, new carpets, wood smoke, or cleaning agents can trigger wheezing and shortness of breath. Inhaling a variety of allergens such as mold, dust, dust mites, animal dander, or pollens from trees, grasses, and weeds can all trigger asthma. Breathing can become labored, and if not addressed, asthma can develop into a life-threatening condition.

An overgrowth of the common yeast *Candida albicans* in the GI tract can also trigger asthma. I have found that a food elimination diet, especially with the avoidance of dairy and wheat products, has been quite helpful in many of my asthma patients. Intramuscular injections of vitamin B_{12} can also help to reduce asthmatic symptoms, especially in children.

In addition to asthma medications, the following are some of the most important nutrients that you may want to consider:

Highly Recommended:

Vitamin C: 1,000 mg three times per day
Magnesium: 400 mg two times per day
Omega-3 fatty acids: 1,000 mg three times per day

Antioxidant supplements: Two times per day
Vitamin E: 400 IU per day
Vitamin B_6: 200 mg per day

Often Recommended:

Quercetin: 250 mg three times per day
Grape seed extract: 100 mg three times per day
Coenzyme Q_{10}: 50 mg twice per day
Selenium: 200 mcg once or twice per day

Beta-carotene: 25,000–50,000 IU per day
Green tea extract: 200 mg three times per day
Ginkgo biloba: 80 mg three times per day

Health Tip: Quercetin

Quercetin is a specific bioflavonoid that acts an an antihistamine and has anti-inflammatory properties. It works well when combined with vitamin C and can be found in onions, tomatoes, green peppers, broccoli, tea, and apples. As a supplement, quercetin has been used to reduce allergy symptoms and to protect LDL cholesterol from damage by free radicals. It may also reduce the risk of diabetic complications.

Health Tip: Grape Seed Extract

Grape seed extract is extremely high in flavonoids and has strong antioxidant and anti-inflammatory effects. It is also high in proanthocyanidins (PCOs), which help to scavenge free radicals. Pycnogenol®, a substance derived from the bark of the French Maritime pine tree, is also high in PCOs and has properties similar to grape seed extract.

Attention Deficit Disorder

Attention deficit disorder (ADD) can occur with or without hyperactivity. ADD has been a term applied to children who have a short attention span, difficulty learning, difficulty paying attention, symptoms of impulsivity (i.e., jumping up and down in class or acting out before giving appropriate thought), emotional instability, or perceptual motor impairment.

In many cases, I have found that food allergies play an important role in ADD. In addition, children with ADD may have been on numerous antibiotics for frequent ear infections and may have an overgrowth of intestinal yeast, *Candida albicans*, in their GI tract. In this regard, it's important that children with ADD avoid simple sugars, caffeine, food additives, artificial flavors, colorings, and preservatives and follow an elimination diet before being treated with any pharmaceutical agents. The following nutrients may be of great value:

Highly Recommended:

Multivitamin and mineral supplement
Vitamin B_6: 50 mg two times per day
Niacinamide: 250 mg two times per day

Vitamin B complex: 50 mg per day
Calcium: 500–1,000 mg per day
Magnesium: 200–400 mg per day

Often Recommended:

GABA: 500 mg three times per day
Zinc: 30–50 mg per day
Inositol: 250 mg two or three times per day

Flaxseed oil: $^1/_2$–1 tablespoon per day
Phosphatidylserine: 100 mg two times per day

Bladder Infections

Bladder infections occur much more frequently in women than in men. They are often caused by bacterial infections that travel up the urethra and into the bladder. Bladder infections can cause urinary frequency, urinary pain or burning, and low-grade fevers. Drinking large quantities of water is certainly recommended and it may be important to have your physician perform a urinalysis and urinary culture. Although doctors frequently prescribe antibiotics for bladder infection, I have found that the following therapies may also be helpful:

Highly Recommended:

Cranberry juice: 16 oz per day
Uva ursi capsules: 300 mg three times per day

Goldenseal: 500 mg two times per day
Vitamin C: 500 mg three times per day

Often Recommended:

Zinc: 30 mg per day
Bioflavonoids: 500 mg two times per day

Vitamin A: 25,000 IU per day

Health Tip: Vitamin A

In high doses, vitamin A can cause headaches or joint and bone pain. During pregnancy, women should not take more than 10,000 IU per day.

Boils

A boil is an inflamed, infected hair follicle that can fill the skin area with pus. They are frequently caused by friction, pressure, or moisture from ill-fitting clothing, which allows the bacteria, *Staphylococcus aureus*, to get under the skin and settle into a hair follicle. Boils frequently form in moist areas such as the armpits or groin or in the back of the neck. Try warm compresses every few hours on the infected area along with taking the following supplements:

Highly Recommended:

Zinc: 30–50 mg one or two times per day
Vitamin A: 10,000 IU per day

Tea tree oil: Applied topically two times per day

Bursitis

Bursitis is caused by inflammation of the fluid-filled sac or bursa that fits between two bones such as the shoulder. Discomfort or pain often results with movement. You might find the following to be helpful:

Highly Recommended:

Intramuscular B_{12} injections: Administered by your physician
Boswellia capsules: 150–400 mg three times per day
Boswellia cream: Apply topically two times per day

Ginger capsules: 250 mg three times per day
Capsaicin ointment: Apply topically two times per day
Bromelain: 500 mg three times per day

Health Tip: Boswellia

Boswellia is an ancient Indian Ayurvedic substance that has anti-inflammatory effects similar to those of nonsteroidal, anti-inflammatory drugs (NSAIDs). In contrast, however, Boswellia does not lead to ulceration of the stomach or gastrointestinal irritation so often seen with NSAIDs.

Candida Overgrowth

As discussed earlier, *Candida albicans* is a fungal organism that can flourish if you are taking antibiotics, birth control pills, or steroid medications, or are consuming a high-sugar diet. In addition to a low-yeast diet and antifungal prescription medications, the following nutrients may also be effective:

Highly Recommended:

Probiotics (acidophilus and bifidobacterium): 5–10 billion units per day

Caprylic acid: Two to four 350 mg capsules per day

Oil of oregano: One to three drops per day

Vitamin C: 500 mg two times per day

Garlic: 500 mg two times per day

Goldenseal: One 250 mg capsule three times per day

Biotin: One to three mg per day

Olive leaf extract: One 250 mg capsule two times per day

Health Tip: Probiotics

Probiotics are a classification of naturally occurring intestinal bacteria beneficial to the integrity of the gut mucosa. Two of the more popular and effective organisms, acidophilus and bifidobacterium, are available in both powder or capsules. Remember to refrigerate them upon purchase.

Health Tip: Caprylic Acid

Caprylic acid is a short-chain fatty acid that has antifungal properties. It can be effective in treating yeast overgrowth in the intestinal tract.

Health Tip: Oil of Oregano

Oil of oregano is an ancient herb that has potent antibacterial, antiviral, antiparasitic, and antifungal properties. For this reason, you may find it to be effective in reducing yeast overgrowth.

Often Recommended:

Flaxseed oil: 1 tablespoon per day

Lipotropic factors: One capsule two times per day

Silymarin: One 150 mg capsule two times per day

Pau D'Arco: One 500 mg capsule twice per day

Health Tip: Pau D'Arco

Pau D'Arco trees are native to Central and South America, and the herb has active constituents that have powerful anti-yeast properties.

Canker Sores

Canker sores are painful mouth ulcers that can occur and recur either individually or in clusters. They result from poor fitting dentures, braces, or trauma from your toothbrush. The following supplements may help to provide relief:

Highly Recommended:

Deglycyrrhizinated licorice (DGL): Chew two 380 mg tablets three times per day or mix 200 mg of powdered DGL in 6 ounces of water. Swish and spit out.

Echinacea: Swish ½–1 teaspoon then swallow three times per day.

Chamomile tincture: Swish 30 drops then swallow two times per day.

Vitamin B complex: 50 mg one or two times per day.

Lactobacillus acidophilus and *bulgaricus*: Chew three tablets (1–2 billion organisms each) three times per day.

Health Tip: Deglycyrrhizinated Licorice (DGL)

Deglycyrrhizinated licorice helps to support the gastrointestinal tract and has been used to help heal duodenal ulcers. This form is free of glycyrrhizin and will not elevate blood pressure. You may be able to reduce the duration of canker sores by chewing DGL tablets.

Health Tip: Chamomile

Chamomile is an herb that is soothing and healing to the oral cavity and gastrointestinal tract. Although it has commonly been used for colic and teething, it may provide some pain relief from canker sores.

Often Recommended:

Quercetin: 500 mg three times per day

Vitamin C: 1,000 mg per day

Cardiovascular Disease

Cardiovascular disease remains the leading cause of death in the United States. If coronary vessels become clogged with excessive amounts of plaque, blood flow may become obstructed, causing the heart to receive insufficient quantities of oxygen. This can lead to chest pain, shortness of breath, palpitations, and fainting spells. High blood pressure, or hypertension, continues to be an extremely common form of cardiovascular disease. If left unchecked, hypertension can cause complications ranging from headaches, dizziness, rapid heart rate, sweating, kidney problems, and retinopathy to stroke, heart attack, and heart failure. Other types of cardiovascular disease include congestive heart failure, valvular heart disease, and irregular heart rhythms.

Despite significant preventive measures and new technologies for diagnosis and treatment, cardiovascular disease remains a serious problem. However, there are many measures that you can take to help reduce your risks. Maintaining your ideal body weight, eliminating cigarette smoking, controlling cholesterol levels and blood pressure, reducing your stress levels, and being physically and mentally active are some lifestyle modifications which can help you reduce the risk of developing vascular disease.

Switching to a low-fat diet based on wholesome foods that are loaded with antioxidants, phytonutrients, and fiber is imperative in combating cardiovascular disease. However, a diet change alone may not be sufficient to rid arteries of plaque buildup.

Recent scientific research has indicated that nutrients play a vital role in the prevention and treatment of cardiovascular disease. Coenzyme Q_{10} has been shown to increase oxygenation to the heart muscle, and can be very effective in preventing heart attacks and congestive heart failure while reducing angina attacks and improving exercise tolerance. Antioxidants such as vitamins E and C play a major role in protecting the heart and reducing the risk of coronary heart disease. The herbs hawthorn, cayenne, and ginger may also benefit cardiac function. While hawthorn can help to relax blood vessels, reduce blood pressure, and improve blood flow, ginger has anti-inflammatory effects. There is now evidence indicating that inflammation and perhaps even viruses and bacteria may also be contributing factors for developing heart disease. Lecithin is valuable in that it acts as a fat emulsifier, and may reduce triglyceride and cholesterol levels. L-carnitine increases oxygen uptake into the mitochondria of cells and allows for better utilization of fat. Garlic has been helpful in lowering blood pressure, and in some cases has been shown to lower cholesterol and triglyceride levels. Gingko biloba, magnesium, and essential fatty acids also play a protective role. Recently, the B vitamins, B_6 and B_{12}, and folic acid have also been found to reduce your risk of cardiovascular disease by lowering levels of the blood protein, homcysteine, which when elevated, can cause premature and accelerated plaque formation.

After supervising more than 50,000 chelation therapy treatments in my office, I continue to be impressed with the effectiveness of this treatment. I have found it to be a wonderful preventive measure as well as a treatment that has reversed vascular disease in thousands of patients. Furthermore, the need for medications is often greatly reduced and frequently completely eliminated.

I have found the following nutrients beneficial for those persons diagnosed with cardiovascular disease:

Highly Recommended:

Coenzyme Q_{10}: 100–200 mg per day

Magnesium: 400 mg two times per day

Vitamin E: 400 IU per day

Vitamin C: 1,000 mg three times per day

Hawthorn: 240 mg two times per day

L-carnitine: 1,000 mg two times per day

Ginkgo biloba: 80 mg three times per day

Beta-carotene: 25,000 IU per day

Alpha-Lipoic acid: 100 mg two times per day

Often Recommended:

Garlic: 1,600–3,200 mg per day

Pantethine: 300 mg three times per day

Folic acid: 1 mg per day

Vitamin B_6: 50 mg two times per day

Vitamin B_{12}: 2,000 mcg per day

Vitamin B_1: 100 mg per day

Chromium: 200 mcg per day

Selenium: 200 mcg per day

Bromelain: 500 mg per day

Ginger: 100 mg per day

Taurine: 500 mg two times per day

Arginine: 500 mg two times per day

Lysine: 500 mg two times per day

Proline: 500 mg two times per day

Green tea extract: 100 mg three times per day

Soy isoflavones: 1,000 mg three times per day

Health Tip: Soy Isoflavones

The compounds in soy, known as isoflavones, have strong antioxidant and immune-enhancing properties. The isoflavones genistein and daidzein have been associated with reducing the risk for developing cancer. They also have a beneficial effect in promoting a healthy cardiovascular system and benefiting cholesterol metabolism. Furthermore, they have been useful in preventing osteoporosis and helping to build strong bones.

Carpal Tunnel Syndrome

Carpal tunnel syndrome involves pain and inflammation caused by compression of the median nerve as it travels down the arm and into the wrist. It can cause discomfort, weakness, difficulty grasping or gripping objects, as well as tingling and burning sensations. Discomfort from carpal tunnel syndrome more frequently occurs in the evening and commonly affects people who perform repetitive or strenuous motions with their hands or wrists. It is more commonly seen in office workers, computer users, or carpenters. Some nutrients you should consider include:

Highly Recommended:

Vitamin B complex: 50 mg per day
Vitamin B_6: 100 mg three times per day

Riboflavin (B_2): 50 mg per day
Pyridoxal-5-phosphate: 50 mg two times per day

Health Tip: Pyridoxal-5-Phosphate

Pyridoxal-5-phosphate is an active form of vitamin B_6. I often use this in combination with vitamin B_6 when treating carpal tunnel syndrome.

Often Recommended:

Bromelain: 500 mg two times per day   Acupuncture

Cataracts

Cataracts frequently occur with advancing age due to a loss of transparency of the lens of the eye. They can begin to cause blurred vision and clouding of the lens. Cataracts can impair your vision and are the leading cause of blindness in the United States, making cataract surgery the most common surgical procedure performed here each year. The lens of the eye is particularly susceptible to free radical damage, and therefore, antioxidant therapy may be of great value. The following are some of the nutrients you might want to consider:

Highly Recommended:

Vitamin C: 1,000 mg two times per day
Vitamin E: 400 IU per day
Selenium: 200 mcg per day

Bilberry: 80 mg three times per day
Zinc: 50 mg per day

Often Recommended:

Glutathione: 250 mg twice per day
Ginkgo biloba: 180–240 mg per day
Lipoic acid: 100 mg per day
Lutein: 20 mg per day
Beta-carotene: 25,000 IU per day

Health Tip: Lutein

Lutein is an antioxidant that is a member of the carotenoid family. It can be found in spinach, leeks, collard greens, peas, kale, and romaine lettuce. It helps to protect the retina of the eye from the damages of sunlight and has been associated with protection from age-related macular degeneration, the leading cause of blindness in people over the age of sixty-five.

Cervical Dysplasia

Cervical dysplasia is a precancerous lesion of the cervix in which abnormal cells are found in a Pap smear. If left untreated, it can progress to cancer. Try to optimize your intake of cruciferous vegetables such as broccoli, Brussels sprouts, and cabbage, as well as foods containing vitamin C, beta-carotene, and folic acid if you have been diagnosed with cervical dysplasia. Risk factors for cervical dysplasia include intercourse before the age of eighteen, cigarette smoking, multiple sex partners, exposure to the human papilloma virus (HPV), and long-term use of birth control pills. Some supplements have been found to be beneficial in this condition:

Highly Recommended:

Folic acid: 5–10 mg per day (available
  through a compounding pharmacy)
Vitamin C: 1,000 mg twice per day

Beta-carotene: 25,000–50,000 units
  per day
Selenium: 200–400 mcg per day

Often Recommended:

Vitamin B$_6$: 50 mg per day

Vitamin B$_{12}$: 1,000 mcg per day

Vitamin A: 25,000 IU per day

Cholesterol

Cholesterol is a fatty, waxy substance that can accumulate in your arteries and lead to plaque formation, thereby obstructing blood flow in your body. As cholesterol is deposited and hardened, a condition known as atherosclerosis, or hardening of the arteries, forms which can be a contributing factor to heart disease.

One lifestyle change that can help lower your cholesterol includes increasing the amount of total fiber in your diet to at least 20–30 grams per day. I also suggest that you maintain your ideal body weight. Reducing the total fat, and especially saturated fat, in your diet is quite helpful. Along with an appropriate weight-loss program, should you need one, regular exercise is an excellent way to lower your cholesterol level and keep it low. Before taking medications to lower your cholesterol level, you should probably consider the following options:

Highly Recommended:

Niacin (as inositol hexaniacinate): This form generally does not cause flushing. Start with 500 mg three times per day with meals and gradually increase to a total of 3,000 mg per day. High doses of other forms of niacin might cause a flushing sensation, temporary itching and redness of the neck, face, and extremities.

Vitamin C: 1,000 mg two times per day

Garlic: 2,000–3,000 mg per day

Gugulipid: 100–200 mg per day

Lecithin granules: 1 tablespoon two times per day

Pantethine: 600–1,200 mg per day

Red yeast rice: 1,200 mg two times per day

Tocotrienols: 25 mg capsules, one or two times per day

Health Tip: Gugulipid

Gugulipid is derived from a thorny tree that is commonly found in India. This Ayurvedic herb has been used to lower cholesterol and triglyceride levels and may reduce the stickiness of platelets. Gugulipid should be used with caution in people with liver disease, inflammatory bowel disease, or diarrhea. Some have reported mild abdominal discomfort when using this extract.

Health Tip: Pantethine

Pantethine is the active form of pantothenic acid that may help to reduce total cholesterol levels and increase HDL.

Health Tip: Red Yeast Rice

Red yeast rice is a traditional Chinese medicine that contains naturally occurring HMG-CoA reductase inhibitors that have been found to raise the "good" HDL cholesterol and lower the "bad" LDL cholesterol as well as total cholesterol. Although some people have reported mild gastrointestinal distress and headaches from this substance, I have generally found it to be an effective alternative to conventional cholesterol-lowering statin drugs.

Often Recommended:

Flaxseed oil: 1 tablespoon per day

Borage oil: 1,200–2,400 mg per day

Chromium picolinate: 200–400 mcg per day

Chronic Fatigue Syndrome

Chronic fatigue syndrome (CFS) is characterized by debilitating fatigue along with a group of other symptoms including a mild fever, recurrent sore throat, swollen and painful lymph nodes, muscle weakness, muscle or joint pain, recurrent headaches, depression, sleep disturbances, and prolonged fatigue after exercise. With chronic fatigue syndrome, your immune system is thought to be impaired, making it difficult to ward off invading viruses, yeast, or bacteria. People with this condition often notice a sudden onset of flu-like symptoms with a significant drop in energy soon thereafter. Subsequently, they begin to complain of brain fog, difficulty with mental functioning, and muscle aches and pains.

At the Magaziner Center for Wellness and Anti-Aging Medicine, I have found that intravenous vitamin and mineral treatments can be extremely valuable in reducing symptoms of CFS. Since there is no specific drug to treat this condition, you might want to consider some of the following nutritional supplements:

Highly Recommended:

Vitamin C: 2,000–4,000 mg per day

Magnesium: 400–800 mg per day

Malic acid: 300–900 mg per day

Vitamin E: 400 IU per day

Coenzyme Q_{10}: 60–200 mg per day

Pantothenic acid: 500 mg twice per day

Health Tip: Malic Acid

Malic acid is a component of the all-important Krebs cycle. Along with magnesium, it can help to generate ATP to improve cellular energy production.

Often Recommended:

NADH: 5 mg two times per day
Siberian ginseng: 100–200 mg per day

Raw adrenal: 1 capsule two times per day
Flaxseed oil: 1 tablespoon per day

Common Cold

The common cold is usually caused by a virus that can affect the upper respiratory tract and cause a sore throat, runny nose, nasal congestion, and general malaise. Although I would recommend extra rest, plenty of fluids, and avoiding eating simple sugars (since they can depress the immune system) you might find that the following treatments also are helpful:

Highly Recommended:

Vitamin C: 1,000 mg three times per day
Zinc lozenges: 23 mg four times per day
Echinacea: 500–1,000 mg per day or $1/2$–1 teaspoon of the tincture or fluid extract per day
Beta-carotene: 50,000–100,000 IU per day

Elderberry: 250 mg capsules or 5–10 ml of the liquid extract twice per day
Goldenseal: 250 mg three times per day
Astragalus: 250 mg capsules or $1/2$–1 teaspoon of tincture three times per day

Health Tip: Elderberry

Elderberry is an herb that contains the flavonoid quercetin. I have found it to be useful in the treatment of the common cold, sore throat, and influenza.

Health Tip: Astragalus

Astragalus is a traditional Chinese herb which contains numerous components to enhance the immune response. It can be useful if you are troubled with frequent colds or sore throats.

Congestive Heart Failure

Congestive heart failure can result when the heart muscle is weakened so much that it cannot effectively pump blood to the rest of the body. As a result, fluids can build up in the lungs and legs. Symptoms can include shortness of breath, fatigue, and inappropriate weight gain. The following nutrients may play a protective role in warding off this serious condition:

Highly Recommended:

Coenzyme Q$_{10}$: 100–400 mg per day

Taurine: 1,000–2,000 mg per day

L-carnitine: 1,000–3,000 mg per day

Hawthorn: 250–500 mg per day

Magnesium: 400–1,200 mg per day

Vitamin E: 400–800 IU per day

Often Recommended:

Thiamine (B$_1$): 100–200 mg per day

Pantethine: 600–1,200 mg per day

Ginkgo biloba: 180–240 mg per day

Arginine: 500–1,000 mg per day

Constipation

Constipation, which occurs when your bowels are not emptying quickly enough, can be a painful and unhealthy condition. When constipated, you retain toxins from your food residues and may feel unwell as a result. Try to increase your intake of fibrous foods such as fresh vegetables, fruit, and whole grains. It is also important to drink at least eight glasses of water with freshly squeezed lemon each day. Regular exercise can increase the muscle contractions in the intestinal tract and help your bowels to move more freely. The following substances can be of great importance:

Highly Recommended:

Beneficial bacteria including acidophilus and bifidobacterium: 3 billion organisms per day

Magnesium: 400 mg per day

Flaxseed oil: 1 tablespoon per day

Psyllium husks: 1 tablespoon in 10 ounces of water or juice per day

Vitamin C: 1,000 mg per day

Health Tip: Psyllium

Psyllium is a bulk-forming laxative high in both fiber and mucilage. It is effective in keeping the feces well hydrated and soft. It is important to drink plenty of water when using psyllium. It has also been effective in cases of high cholesterol and diabetes.

Often Recommended:

Chlorophyll: 50 mg three times per day   Triphala: 500 mg two times per day
Senna: 10 mg per day

Health Tip: Chlorophyll

Chlorophyll is the substance that makes plants green. It has been used to reduce the odors found in halitosis, bad breath, as well as in stool and feces. It is found in dark green leafy vegetables. Chlorophyll supplements may help in reducing both halitosis and constipation.

Health Tip: Senna

Senna grows as a shrub in India, Pakistan, and China. As an herb, it stimulates the activity of the colon and assists with bowel movements. It, therefore, can be used for constipation but should not be used for more than ten days at a time nor in children under age six. Long-term use of senna can cause your colon to become dependent on it in order to effectively move your bowels.

Health Tip: Triphala

Triphala is an Indian Ayurvedic herb made up of a mixture of equal proportions of the dried fruits of three plants and has been helpful for constipation. It is best taken before bedtime.

Crohn's Disease

Crohn's disease is an inflammatory bowel disorder that can cause bloody diarrhea and malabsorption. Crohn's disease frequently affects the last part of the small intestine. I would certainly recommend the elimination of food allergies and reduction of sugar intake. Many persons have also responded favorably to reducing dairy and wheat intake. Several nutrients may help in reducing your symptoms of Crohn's disease. These include the following:

Highly Recommended:

Pantothenic acid: 500 mg twice per day

Fish oil capsules: 1,000 mg three times per day

Pantethine: 300 mg twice per day

Multiple vitamin and minerals

Vitamin E: 400 IU per day

Vitamin C: 1,000 mg two times per day

Zinc: 30 mg two times per day

Often Recommended:

Vitamin A: 25,000 IU per day

Slippery elm: 350 mg capsule or 1 teaspoon as a tincture three times per day

Marshmallow root: 450 mg three times per day

Fresh cabbage juice: 4 ounces per day

Health Tip: Slippery Elm

The slippery elm tree is native to North America. As an herbal supplement, slippery elm can be taken internally for digestive disorders and sore throat. It is soothing to the GI tract and I have found it useful in cases of Crohn's disease. It is also used as an ingredient in throat lozenges or cough drops.

Health Tip: Marshmallow Root

Marshmallow root is soothing and healing to the digestive tract and inflamed mucous membranes. It can also be effective as a tea or as a tincture by using one to two teaspoons three times per day.

Depression

People with depression become withdrawn, have difficulty experiencing pleasure, and lose interest in many of their prior activities. They sometimes complain of excessive fatigue, insomnia, nervousness, poor appetite, low libido, mood swings, and feelings of inadequacy. Other symptoms include feelings of guilt, worthlessness, difficulty in concentrating and making decisions, restlessness, irritability, persistent feelings of sadness, emptiness, hopelessness, helplessness, and pessimism. Hereditary factors often play a role. Nearly half of those with depression, for instance, state that one or both of their parents had similar symptoms.

Metabolic imbalances can contribute to depression. A full assessment of trace minerals and vitamins—especially B_{12}, folic acid, and amino acids—is especially helpful here. It is also important to rule out a weak adrenal gland, hypoglycemia, cancer, liver disease, kidney problems, hypothyroidism, menopausal syndrome, and food allergies when dealing with depression.

Also associated with causing depression is an imbalance in the body's supply of neurotransmitters such as serotonin. These neurotransmitters are responsible for carrying messages for hunger, thirst, anger, memory, alertness, and sleepiness as well as depression, anxiety, panic attacks, and obsessive compulsive behavior. This has led to the development of new prescription antidepressants, all of which are associated with many side effects. As a result, I almost always first try to treat depression with natural therapies, dietary changes, exercise, and lifestyle modifications before resorting to pharmaceuticals.

Other helpful lifestyle changes include avoiding sugar and simple carbohydrates, which can increase fatigue and depression, and avoiding alcohol and caffeine. At the same time, try to eat more complex carbohydrates, especially those from fresh fruit, vegetables, whole grains, and beans, along with protein derived from lean meats, fish, and chicken. This will help to boost your serotonin levels, which can reduce your depression. Normal rest and natural sunlight can lessen feelings of depression as well.

Of the nutritional supplements that have been shown to reduce depressive symptoms, I suggest the following:

Highly Recommended:

Vitamin B complex: 50 mg per day
Vitamin B_{12}: 1,000–2,000 mcg per day
St. John's wort: 300 mg three times per day

Tyrosine: 500 mg two times per day
SAMe: 400–800 mg per day
5-Hydroxytryptophan (5-HTP): 100 mg three times per day

Health Tip: SAMe

SAMe (S-adenosyl-methionine) has been useful to improve joint health and mood. I have found it useful in the treatment of osteoarthritis, fibromyalgia, and depression. SAMe may also help normalize liver function in patients with hepatitis or cirrhosis. It is best absorbed when taken on an empty stomach.

Often Recommended:

Phosphatidylserine: 300 mg per day
Inositol: 3,000–9,000 mg per day
Vitamin B_6: 100 mg two times per day

Niacinamide: 500–1000 mg per day
NADH: 5–10 mg per day
Ginkgo biloba: 60 mg two times per day

Diabetes Mellitus

Diabetes is a condition that causes inappropriate sugar metabolism. Common symptoms include increased thirst, frequent urination, excessive hunger, blurred vision, poor circulation, or numbness and tingling in the feet or lower extremities.

There are more than 10 million Americans who are currently being treated for diabetes. Juvenile diabetes, which occurs before the age of thirty, is the result of insufficient amounts of insulin in the blood. Juvenile diabetes is frequently responsive to insulin injections—insulin being necessary to metabolize blood sugar and store it in muscle, where it's used later for energy. Adult-onset diabetes usually occurs after age thirty and is more responsive to dietary changes, exercise, weight loss, and nutritional supplements. In adult-onset diabetes, although the pancreas generally secretes adequate amounts of insulin, the body has grown resistant to it, rendering it ineffective. Hereditary factors often play a role.

Many people with adult-onset diabetes are obese. For them, diabetes treatment includes weight loss to help reduce blood sugar. Regular exercise can improve insulin secretion from the pancreas and insulin utilization, reduce fatigue, and promote weight loss. To reduce the need for insulin, strive to consume a diet low in saturated fats and simple sugars, and high in fiber and complex carbohydrates. Various legumes, vegetables, and whole grains are particularly valuable. Many diabetics must also avoid consuming large quantities of fruit, fruit juices, or starchy carbohydrates.

Some diabetics are deficient in trace minerals, chromium, zinc, manganese, and magnesium. These individuals seem to respond well to supplements to help reduce their need for diabetic medications or insulin injections. B-complex vitamins and antioxidants are particularly effective in assisting diabetics in controlling symptoms. Other supplements to consider include vitamin C with bioflavonoids, biotin, and vitamin E, as well as herbal remedies such as bilberry and gymnema sylvestre. Since long-term diabetes can contribute to neuropathy or numbness and tingling in the extremities, supplemental evening primrose oil, alpha-lipoic acid, and inositol are recommended.

Although there are numerous medications and insulin injections available to help control diabetes, I have found the following supplements beneficial:

Highly Recommended:

Chromium picolinate: 200 mcg two to four times per day

Vitamin E: 400 IU two times per day

Vitamin C: 100 mg two times per day

Alpha-lipoic acid: 100–200 mg per day

Gymnema sylvestrae: 400 mg per day

Vitamin B complex: 50 mg per day

Bioflavonoids: 1,000 mg two times per day

Magnesium: 400 mg per day

Vitamin B_6: 50 mg two times per day

Zinc: 30 mg per day

Evening primrose oil: 500 mg two times per day

Health Tip: Gymnema sylvestrae

The leaves of the gymnema sylvestrae, which grow in India, have a strong blood sugar–lowering effect. It has been useful in the treatment of diabetes and helps to raise insulin levels. I have also found that gymnema sylvestrae can help lower both cholesterol and triglyceride levels. Although it is generally very safe, diabetics should use gymnema only under the supervision of a health-care professional.

Often Recommended:

Biotin: 1 mg two times per day
Coenzyme Q_{10}: 50 mg two times per day
Inositol: 500 mg two times per day
L-carnitine: 500 mg two times per day

Ginkgo biloba: 40 mg three times per day
Fiber: 20–30 mg per day
Flaxseed oil: 1 tablespoon per day
Bilberry: 80 mg two times per day

Digestive Difficulties

More and more Americans complain of problems with digestion and assimilation each year. Common symptoms include excessive intestinal gas, bloating, cramping, heartburn, diarrhea and constipation. Although digestive problems come from many sources, the most frequently cited include food allergies, which may exacerbate digestive symptoms; abnormal intestinal bacteria and yeast overgrowth, which usually occur after a course of antibiotics or by consuming contaminated food and water; inadequate production of hydrochloric acid, which leads to excessive gas and bloating and may affect your ability to absorb nutrients from food; and an inadequate secretion of pancreatic enzymes, which may prevent you from digesting or assimilating your food properly.

Natural therapies are wide-ranging and quite beneficial. For example, supplemental digestive enzymes along with the good intestinal bacteria, such as *Lactobacillus acidophilus* and *bifidus,* can assist in digestion and assimilation. Pancreatic enzymes, such as protease, amylase, and lipase, are also valuable as digestive aids. Glutamine, an important metabolic fuel for cells lining the intestinal walls, can help in absorbing nutrients and in preventing muscle loss. Papaya and bromelain, an enzyme derived from pineapple, also reduce intestinal gas and bloating.

Because intestinal gas and bloating can also be caused by consuming inadequate amounts of fiber or simply by eating too many processed and refined foods, you may find that proper food combining can also lessen your symptoms.

If you have digestive difficulties, the following recommendations will be of help:

Highly Recommended:

Beneficial bacteria (probiotics): $^1\!/_2$–1 teaspoon per day

Fiber: 5 grams per day

Pancreatic enzymes: One dose at the end of each meal

Glutamine: 500 mg two times per day

Peppermint oil capsules (enteric coated): One or two between meals

Often Recommended:

Bromelain: 500 mg after meals

Papaya: 1–2 tablets after each meal

Dupuytren's Contracture

In Dupuytren's contracture, fibrous tissue forms in the palm of the hand which can lead to the fingers curling up toward the palm. Although surgery may be required in more severe cases, you may want to first try:

Highly Recommended:

Vitamin E: 400 IU two times per day by mouth and topical vitamin E oil

Ear Infections

Chronic ear infections frequently affect children under the age of five. They are most commonly treated with antibiotics, and if they persist, ear tubes may be inserted surgically. Ear infections account for approximately 50 percent of all visits to pediatricians. Although antibiotics are the most common therapy recommended, there are other kinds of preventative treatments available. Elimination of food allergens can be very helpful and the avoidance of dairy products should be considered. Various environmental factors such as a wood-burning stove or being exposed to secondhand smoke can also trigger ear infections. Infants who are breastfed have a lower risk for recurrent ear infections. Some selective nutrients may be helpful in reducing the frequency of ear infections:

Highly Recommended:

Vitamin C: 250–1,000 mg per day, depending on age

Vitamin A: 25,000–50,000 IU per day up to 5–7 days

Beta-carotene: 10,000–100,000 IU per day, depending on age

Zinc: 5–25 mg per day

Often Recommended:

Bioflavonoids: 100–500 mg per day

Echinacea: 325–650 mg per day if freeze-dried, or ½–1 teaspoon of tincture or fluid extract

Mullein oil drops inserted into the ear canal

Health Tip: Mullein Oil

Mullein oil has been used as a remedy for the respiratory tract, particularly in cases of chronic congestion, bronchitis, cough, and even for asthma and pneumonia. It has a soothing effect on the mucous membranes, and for this reason, drops can be placed in the ears for earaches or ear pain. For pulmonary conditions, I recommend ½–1 teaspoon of tincture by mouth two or three times per day.

Eczema

Eczema is a common condition in which the skin is very dry, itchy, inflamed, thickened, red, and frequently scaly. Most people with eczema have either food or inhalant allergies that worsen their condition. Eczema frequently affects the face, wrists, elbows, and knees. You might want to try an elimination diet that avoids milk and dairy products, eggs, tomatoes, peanuts, and artificial colors or preservatives for at least two months. Try to eat more fatty fish such as salmon, mackerel, cod, herring, and halibut. If you have taken antibiotics on a frequent basis, an overgrowth of intestinal yeast may also contribute to your eczema. Several nutritional supplements may be of benefit, which can include the following:

Highly Recommended:

Omega-3 oils, such as fish oils or flaxseed oil: 5–10 grams per day
Vitamin E: 400 IU per day

Zinc: 30–60 mg per day
Vitamin C: 1,000 mg two times per day
Quercetin: 100 mg per day

Often Recommended:

Evening primrose oil: 3,000 mg per day
Grape seed extract: 100 mg two times per day

Licorice root: As a tincture, $^1/_2$–1 teaspoon three times per day, or applied topically three times per day

Health Tip: Licorice Root

Licorice root reduces the inflammation and itching that is associated with eczema. It can be taken either orally or used topically to alleviate symptoms. The soothing action of licorice is also useful in reducing cough and sore throat symptoms. People with hypertension, however, should avoid using licorice long term, unless the glycyrrhizin (a substance in licorice that elevates blood pressure) has been removed.

Fatigue

Overwhelming fatigue has recently grown into a common complaint heard by doctors across the country. Common causes are quite varied and include anemia, hypothyroidism, reactive hypoglycemia, adrenal insufficiency, cancer, lack of exercise, depression, a diet of devitalized food, excessive stress, yeast overgrowth, insomnia, viral or bacterial illness, allergies, and exposure to environmental toxins. Cigarette smoking, excessive alcohol intake, and various medications may also contribute to fatigue.

While we need to evaluate and treat the biochemical, metabolic, and psychosocial causes of fatigue, a sound nutritional program is vital. A diet of wholesome foods over the so-called "energy robbers"—like soft drinks, refined and processed foods, and sweets and desserts—is essential in combating fatigue. Fresh fruit and vegetables, whole grains, nuts and seeds, and fish or lean meats will help provide the fuel you need as well. Getting proper rest (at least eight hours of sleep per night), fresh air, stretching and exercising on a regular basis, being exposed to natural sunlight, having a happy relationship with a spouse or a loved one, and maintaining a positive attitude can all go a long way in lifting fatigue.

Many people with fatigue have vitamin, mineral, and amino acid, or essential fatty acid imbalances. A sound multivitamin program including trace minerals, magnesium, vitamin B_{12}, folic acid, and pantothenic acid is very helpful. Vitamin C with bioflavonoids, free-form amino acids, vitamin E, and herbs such as ginseng and gotu kola make excellent complements to the program.

If you are tired of feeling so tired, the following substances may be beneficial:

Highly Recommended:

Magnesium: 400 mg per day
Malic acid: 300 mg two times per day
Coenzyme Q_{10}: 60 mg two times per day
NADH: 5 mg two times per day

Vitamin B_{12}: 2,000 mcg per day
Multivitamin with trace minerals
Vitamin C: 1,000 mg two times per day
Bioflavonoids: 500 mg two times per day

Often Recommended:

Vitamin E: 400 IU per day
Adrenal glandular: One tablet two times per day
Gotu kola: 60 mg one or two times per day

Siberian ginseng: 250 mg two times per day
Vitamin B complex: 50 mg per day

Health Tip: Gotu Kola

Gotu kola has been used in Central Asia for medicinal purposes for many years. It can be helpful in boosting cognitive function and mental clarity and may be useful in chronic fatigue.

Fibrocystic Breast Disease

Fibrocystic breast disease is a common condition frequently affecting younger woman when their breasts become tender, painful, or lumpy. This condition is generally considered to be benign and may worsen premenstrually. Many women have found that the elimination of caffeine can greatly reduce their symptoms. Be aware that caffeine can be found not only in coffee but also in most teas, cola drinks, chocolate, and numerous medications. I have found that the following nutrients can be helpful in reducing symptoms of fibrocystic breast disease:

Highly Recommended:

Vitamin E: 400 IU two times per day

Evening primrose oil: 3,000 mg per day

Vitamin B_6: 50 mg two times per day

Often Recommended:

Chasteberry (Vitex agnus cactus): 250 mg of dried, powdered extract or 40 drops of liquid extract per day

Dong quai: 2–3 grams per day

Flaxseed oil: 1 tablespoon per day

Choline: 500 mg per day

Methionine: 500 mg per day

Health Tip: Chasteberry (Vitex agnus cactus)

Vitex agnus cactus can help to normalize hormone balance and alleviate symptoms of PMS. It stimulates the pituitary gland to produce more luteinizing hormone, which then increases progesterone production. It also may be beneficial in treating infertility and fibrocystic breast disease. Vitex is not recommended for pregnant or nursing women.

Health Tip: Dong Quai

Dong quai helps to promote normal hormonal balance and may be helpful in women experiencing menstrual pain, cramping, or uterine bleeding. Some women have found that dong quai reduces symptoms of fibrocystic breast disease as well. Dong quai is not recommended for pregnant or lactating women. Because dong quai can cause sun sensitivity in light-skinned individuals, prolonged exposure to sunlight should be avoided.

Fibromyalgia

Fibromyalgia is a serious disorder characterized by muscle aches or pain, or local stiffness throughout the body. A doctor will usually palpate several points where specific muscles are abnormally tender, usually around the back of the head, neck, shoulders, and back. You may also complain of general fatigue, headaches, insomnia, joint swelling, numbness or tingling sensations, mild depression, or an irritable bowel. Know that your physical activity, stress levels, and changes in the weather can affect all such symptoms.

Because there are no laboratory studies or blood evaluations to confirm whether or not you have fibromyalgia, you must rely on your doctor's clinical acumen for a diagnosis.

Some evidence suggests, however, that fibromyalgia may be associated with autoimmune abnormalities, viral infections such as Epstein-Barr virus, hypothyroidism, chronic mercury exposure from dental amalgam, overgrowth of *Candida albicans,* and chemical sensitivities.

When treating fibromyalgia, appropriate lifestyle changes are essential. Don't smoke cigarettes and avoid the "empty calories" found in white sugar, processed foods, and alcohol. Mild stretching and exercise are excellent adjuncts here.

If you suffer from any of the symptoms just mentioned, get evaluated for vitamin and trace mineral imbalances, and should deficiencies be found, take appropriate nutritional supplements. I frequently suggest also having your amino acids, essential fatty acids, and digestion and assimilation evaluated. Many people with fibromyalgia also suffer from leaky gut syndrome and are not effectively absorbing their nutrients. Supplemental nutrients such as magnesium with malic acid to improve energy production within the muscles, coenzyme Q_{10} to assist in tissue oxygenation, L-carnitine, and vitamin C with bioflavonoids seem extremely effective in dealing with such symptoms. B vitamins, of course, are particularly important for energy utilization and normal brain function. Some people have found that ingesting B vitamins orally helps to reduce symptoms, while others have had a better response to B complex injections with extra vitamin B_{12}. Since fibromyalgia may accelerate the production of free radicals, make antioxidants part of your treatment as well. Supplements with essential fatty acids such as evening primrose oil or flaxseed oil will also help to protect against cell damage and reduce fatigue and pain.

A diet of wholesome foods is very important. Many patients with fibromyalgia are found to have numerous food allergies and sensitivities; thus, avoiding allergenic foods is important for these people. Others have also been diagnosed with mold, inhalant, and chemical allergies. Reducing the "total allergenic load" in fibromyalgia therapy is crucial.

Some of the most frequently helpful nutrients include:

Highly Recommended:

Magnesium: 400 mg two times per day
Malic acid: 800–2,400 mg daily
Vitamin E: 400 IU daily
Vitamin B_1: 100 mg two times per day
Vitamin C: 1,000 mg three times per day

SAMe: 400–1,200 mg per day
High-quality multivitamin with minerals
Vitamin B_{12}: 1,000 mcg per day
Coenzyme Q_{10}: 60 mg three times per day
Zinc: 25 mg two times per day

Often Recommended:

NADH: 2.5 mg two times per day

L-carnitine: 1,000 mg three times per day

5-hydroxy L-tryptophan (5-HTP): 100 mg
three times per day

St. John's wort: 300 mg three times
per day

Gallstones

Gallstones frequently cause pain in the upper right quadrant of the abdomen that may be accompanied with nausea and vomiting. The discomfort is caused by obstruction of the flow of bile from the bile duct due to the gallstones. Although gallstones may occur without any symptoms, more than 300,000 gallbladder surgeries are performed each year in the United States. Women are more susceptible to gallstones than men especially if they are obese.

I have found an elimination diet very helpful in reducing the extent and severity of gallbladder attacks. Attempt to eliminate coffee entirely. You might find a vegetarian diet, high fiber intake, and elimination of refined sugar helpful as well. Try to limit your intake of saturated fats, dietary cholesterol, and fried foods while increasing your intake of water to at least eight glasses per day. In addition, the following nutritional supplements can also provide relief:

Highly Recommended:

Lecithin: 100 mg three times per day

Vitamin C: 1,000 mg two times per day

Vitamin E: 400 IU per day

Choline: 1,000 mg per day

Fiber supplement (such as oat bran,
guar gum, psyllium, or pectin): 5 grams
per day

Often Recommended:

Silymarin (milk thistle): 600 mg per day

Curcumin: 400 mg three times per day

Health Tip: Curcumin

Curcumin, the compound that gives turmeric its yellow color and flavor, is frequently used as a key ingredient in many curries. Curcumin functions as an antioxidant to protect you against free radical damage and can also reduce inflammation. It can protect the liver from toxic compounds and is involved in liver detoxification. Curcumin may also be useful in people with gallstones to assist liver filtration.

Gingivitis

Gingivitis involves inflammation of the gums and is also known as periodontal disease. If left untreated, this problem can cause loss of bone that supports the teeth. You might find the following recommendations helpful:

Highly Recommended:

Coenzyme Q_{10}: 100 mg two times per day
Vitamin C with bioflavonoids: 1,000 mg
two times per day

Folic acid: 0.1% solution to be used as a
mouthwash and 5 mg capsule per day

Often Recommended:

Chamomile: 1 cup of tea two times per day
Echinacea: Apply tincture topically to the gums
Myrrh: Apply the tincture topically to the gums or take 1–2 ml of tincture three times per day

Peppermint: Can drink as a tea or can apply the oil topically to the gums
Massage your gums with a mixture of hydrogen peroxide and baking soda

Health Tip: Myrrh

Myrrh has a soothing effect on inflammation in the mouth and throat. It can be used to treat periodontal disease, gingivitis, canker sores, and sore throats associated with the common cold. The tincture can be applied topically to the gums or canker sores or can be taken orally at a dose of 1–2 ml three times per day.

Health Tip: Peppermint

As a general digestive aid, peppermint is helpful for colic, indigestion, and intestinal cramping. It can be also used topically in cases of gingivitis to reduce pain and irritation.

As a tea, peppermint can be consumed on a regular basis. When used in large amounts, peppermint oil can cause gastrointestinal upset and burning and should probably be avoided if you suffer from chronic heartburn.

Glaucoma

Glaucoma occurs with the buildup of excess pressure within the eye. If left untreated, this condition can lead to blindness. Most often, glaucoma is controlled with the use of eye-drops to help lower intraocular pressure. I have found the following nutritional approaches are also beneficial and free of the possible side effects associated with glaucoma eye drop treatments:

Highly Recommended:

Vitamin C: 5–10 grams per day
Bioflavonoids: 100 mg two times per day
Rutin: 50 mg per day

Flaxseed oil: 1 tablespoon per day
Magnesium: 400 mg per day
Ginkgo biloba: 40 mg three times per day

Health Tip: Rutin

Rutin is a bioflavonoid that may help reduce pressure within the eye and has been a part of my glaucoma treatment for some time.

Often Recommended:

Flaxseed oil: 1 tablespoon per day
Chromium: 200 mcg two times per day

Bilberry: 80 mg three times per day

Hay Fever

Hay fever problems occur when you have allergic reactions to pollens in the air from trees, grasses, or weeds most frequently in the spring or summer. Ragweed pollen accounts for approximately 75 percent of the hay fever problems in the United States. Common symptoms include sneezing, eye irritation, or nasal congestion and mucus production. In lieu of drugs, you might want to consider the following treatments:

Highly Recommended:

Vitamin C: 1,000–3,000 mg per day

Quercetin: 500 mg three times per day

Bioflavonoids: 1,000 mg two times per day

Stinging nettle: 400 mg capsule or ½–1 teaspoon of tincture three times per day

Health Tip: Stinging Nettle

Stinging nettle may help in reducing your symptoms of hay fever including itchy eyes and sneezing. It has also been used successfully to treat the symptoms of benign prostatic hyperplasia (BPH).

Often Recommended:

Ginkgo biloba: 40 mg three times per day   Nasal saline washes

Headaches

Headaches can be caused by numerous factors including food allergies, excessive sugar or caffeine, stress or tension, muscle spasms, or spinal misalignment. Relaxation techniques are quite beneficial in reducing headache discomfort, and you may also find that massage or manipulation are of great benefit. I have found that the following nutrients may also prevent the onset of headaches:

Highly Recommended:

Magnesium: 400 mg two times per day

Vitamin B_6: 25 mg two times per day

Vitamin B complex: 50 mg per day

Vitamin C: 1,000 mg two times per day

Feverfew: 100 mg two times per day

Ginkgo biloba: 240 mg per day

5-Hydroxy L-tryptophan (5-HTP): 100 mg three times per day

Often Recommended:

Ginger: 1 capsule twice per day

Bromelain: 500 mg two times per day

Vitamin E: 400 IU per day

Flaxseed oil: 1 tablespoon per day

Hemorrhoids

Hemorrhoids occur when enlarged or varicosed veins form in the rectal region. When inflamed, they can bleed, often leading to itching and pain. Increasing your intake of fiber especially from psyllium and insoluble fiber from whole grains and vegetables can increase the bulk of the stool and reduce susceptibility to hemorrhoids. I also suggest drinking large quantities of water each day. You may have success in reducing hemorrhoid symptoms by trying the following as well:

Highly Recommended:

Vitamin E suppositories: One at bedtime

Horse chestnut: 250 mg two times per day

Butcher's broom: 1,000 mg capsules two times per day, ointment to be applied topically, or rectal suppositories to be compounded by your local pharmacist

Psyllium fiber: 3–5 grams per day

Health Tip: Butcher's Broom

The herb butcher's broom is derived from a small-leafed evergreen bush native to Northwest Europe and the Mediterranean region. Butcher's broom applied as an ointment or used as a suppository has an anti-inflammatory effect and can help heal hemorrhoids by constricting small veins. Alternatively, capsules of butcher's broom may also be effective.

Often Recommended:

Bioflavonoids: 2,000-4,000 mg per day

Vitamin C: 500 mg two times per day

Rutin: 50 mg two times per day

Hepatitis

Hepatitis involves an inflammation of the liver that can be caused by medications, drugs, or viruses. You can also contract hepatitis from contaminated food, infected blood transfusions, or sexual contact. There are several different types of hepatitis and each of these needs medical attention. Whatever type of hepatitis you have, however, it is important to support the liver, improve immune function, and attempt to regenerate liver cells damaged by the disease. A nutrient-dense diet that is plentiful in high-fiber foods, brown rice, vegetables, and fresh fruit, and has moderate amounts of lean protein is an important adjunct in healing. I also suggest that you minimize your intake of fried foods, saturated fats, and simple carbohydrates including white flour, and sugar. Alcohol, aspirin, acetaminophen, and ibuprofen should be avoided. In order to protect the cells of the liver, you might want to consider the following:

Highly Recommended:

Vitamin C: 2,000 to 8,000 mg per day (Intravenous infusions of vitamin C may also be helpful.)

Silymarin or milk thistle: 400 mg per day
Licorice: 250 mg three times per day
Liver extract: 500–1,000 mg per day

Often Recommended:

Alpha-lipoic acid: 100 mg three times per day
Thymus extracts: 500 mg per day
Choline: 500 mg two times per day

Inositol: 500 mg two times per day
Vitamin B complex: 50 mg per day
Glutathione: 250 mg two times per day

Health Tip: Thymus Extract

Thymus extract can be taken orally to help enhance the function of the immune system. Thymus extract is also helpful in reducing the number of recurrent infections. In cases of hepatitis, thymus extract works to help support the body's general defense.

Health Tip: Glutathione

Glutathione is a potent antioxidant that can protect you from damaging free radicals. As such, it can help protect the liver against environmental toxins and medication residues. Glutathione is actually composed of three amino acids: cysteine, glutamic acid, and glycine. In cases of hepatitis, I frequently combine glutathione with other nutrients to protect the liver from free radical damage.

Hypertension

Hypertension, or high blood pressure, affects millions of people worldwide. In this condition, blood pressure is consistently found to be elevated above 140/90. Because hypertension can be a risk factor for suffering a stroke or a heart attack, lifestyle changes are important therapeutic adjuncts. These include reducing the consumption of coffee, alcohol, cigarette smoking, and reducing stress while increasing physical activity, high-fiber foods, garlic, onions, fresh green vegetables, and fatty fish such as salmon, cod, and mackerel. Many of my patients have been able to reduce blood pressure with lifestyle and dietary modifications, and nutritional supplements, thus avoiding the need for medications and all their related side effects. Some of the most important nutrients include the following:

Highly Recommended:

Fish oils: 2,000 to 4,000 mg per day

Flaxseed oil: 1 tablespoon two times per day

Garlic: 1,800–2,400 mg per day

Coenzyme Q$_{10}$: 100–200 mg per day

Magnesium: 400 mg two times per day

Hawthorn: 250 mg three times per day

Antioxidant formula: Two times per day

Often Recommended:

Vitamin C: 1,000 mg two times per day

Taurine: 1,000 mg two times per day

Green tea: 1 cup per day

Immune Dysfunction

The immune system is a very complicated and intricate network of specialized cells, organs, and chemicals that communicate with each other to help prevent and fight infections and to ward off cancer. If you have a weakened immune system, you may be more prone to colds, flu, and viruses and more susceptible to cancer. A wholesome nutrient-rich diet, adequate rest, and reducing stress can all help to improve your immune response. I also suggest that you limit your intake of white flour, refined and simple sugars, and environmental toxins. In my practice, I have used nutritional supplements to successfully treat thousands of patients who were troubled with a weakened immune system. These supplements include the following:

Highly Recommended:

Vitamin C: 1–3 grams per day

Zinc: 25 mg per day

Echinacea capsules: 250 mg three times per day or 30 drops per day

Garlic: 2,400 mg per day

Green tea: 2 cups per day

Multivitamin with minerals

Often Recommended:

Maitake D-fraction: 50 drops per day or 2 capsules two times per day

Astragalus: 30 drops per day or 250 mg capsules two times per day

Vitamin A: 25,000 IU per day

Vitamin E: 400 IU per day

Goldenseal capsules: Two 250 mg per day

Health Tip: Maitake D-fraction

Extracts of maitake mushrooms are used as supportive treatment in diabetes, cancer, HIV, hypertension, and immune dysfunction. Maitake mushrooms contain active polysaccharides that act as immune enhancers. The D-fraction is the most potent polysaccharide that has been isolated from the maitake mushroom.

Impotence

Impotency is defined as a male's inability to attain and maintain an erection of the penis sufficient enough for sexual intercourse. The majority of impotency cases are related to health conditions such as diabetes or hypertension. Numerous drugs including antihistamines, antidepressants, tranquilizers, antipsychotics, and medications to lower blood pressure have been associated with increasing the risk of impotency. Excessive alcohol consumption and cigarette smoking are also potential risk factors. Although medications and surgical procedures exist that may help to treat impotency, natural therapies may also be effective:

Highly Recommended:

Yohimbine tincture: 15–30 drops per day or 15–30 mg capsules per day

Ginseng: 250 mg two times per day

Vitamin C: 500 mg three times per day

Zinc: 30 mg per day

Muira puama: 250 mg three times per day

Health Tip: Yohimbine

The bark of the yohimbe tree, which grows primarily in Western Africa, has been used to treat male impotency and infertility by dilating blood vessels in the penis. Since it seems to inhibit monoamine oxidase (MAO), foods that are high in tyramine such as cheese, red wine, and liver should be avoided while taking yohimbine; otherwise, it can cause severe hypertension. People with kidney disease as well as women who are pregnant or lactating should also avoid yohimbine. Generally, yohimbine is best taken under the supervision of a doctor.

Health Tip: Muira puama

Muira puama (or potency wood) is an herb that has been used to help treat erectile dysfunction and loss of libido. It appears to boost both the psychological and physical aspects of the sex drive.

Often Recommended:

Ginkgo biloba: 40 mg three times per day   Flaxseed oil: 1 tablespoon per day
Vitamin E: 400 IU per day

Insomnia

Getting a restful night's sleep and feeling refreshed upon awakening in the morning is certainly a key factor in optimal wellness. Insomnia, or difficulty falling asleep, adversely affects millions of people on a regular basis. Although there are many effective prescription and over-the-counter drugs for insomnia, I always suggest trying natural therapies first:

Highly Recommended:

Melatonin: 500–2,500 mcg before bedtime   5-Hydroxy L-trytophan (5-HTP): 100–200
Valerian: 300 mg at bedtime   mg before bedtime

Health Tip: Melatonin

Melatonin, a hormone secreted by the pineal gland located in the brain, helps to regulate sleep and wakefulness. When taken before bedtime, melatonin can be an effective sleep aid. Normal levels of melatonin peak around the age of twenty-five and then begin to decline as you age. This might account for one of the reasons why elderly people can experience difficulty in getting a sound night of sleep.

Often Recommended:

Inositol: 500 mg before bedtime   Magnesium: 400 mg
Look for a combination supplement containing herbs such as chamomile, hops,
  skullcap, or passionflower.

Irritable Bowel Syndrome

Irritable bowel syndrome (IBS) is a common gastrointestinal disorder characterized by excessive gas, bloating, abdominal discomfort, and alternating constipation and diarrhea. Increasing your dietary fiber and avoiding food allergies can both be helpful in reducing IBS symptoms. I also recommend limiting your intake of sweets, refined carbohydrates, and soft drinks. An estimated 15 percent of the population suffers from IBS. The following nutrients may be helpful in reducing your symptoms:

Highly Recommended:

Enteric-coated peppermint oil capsules: 1 capsule three times per day, between meals

Lactobacillus acidophilus: 1–2 billion organisms per day

Evening primrose oil: 1,300 mg per day

Often Recommended:

Fiber supplements: 5 grams per day

Chamomile tea or tincture: ½–1 ml in warm water three times per day

Fennel seeds: Chew ½ teaspoon per day

Health Tip: Fennel Seeds

Fennel seeds are frequently used as a spice when cooking fish and other foods. The seeds can be chewed or used as a tea to help with indigestion, intestinal gas, or irritable bowel syndrome. Pregnant or lactating women, however, should avoid large quantities of fennel seeds.

Kidney Stones

Kidney stones can cause excruciating flank or kidney pain accompanied by nausea, vomiting, chills, fever, and abdominal distention. The most common form of kidney stone is made of calcium oxalate. Dietary recommendations include an increase in dietary fiber, green leafy vegetables and fresh fruit and a decrease in refined carbohydrates, alcohol, fat, and animal protein. I also suggest increasing your intake of foods with a high magnesium to calcium ratio such as rye, soy, buckwheat, corn, barley, oats, brown rice, bananas, peanuts, avocado, coconut, potatoes, sesame seeds, and lima beans. Nutritional supplements frequently help to reduce the recurrence rate of kidney stones, some of which include the following:

Highly Recommended:

Magnesium: 400–800 mg per day
Vitamin B$_6$: 50 mg per day

Potassium citrate: 99 mg three times per day

Often Recommended:

Vitamin K: 2 mg per day
Aloe vera: 1 capsule daily

Cranberry juice: 4 oz per day

Macular Degeneration

Macular degeneration is the leading cause of blindness in the United States in the elderly population. People with macular degeneration have difficulty reading the newspaper or seeing the small print in books and magazines. In my practice, I have seen wonderful results with both intravenous and oral vitamin supplementation. In particular, antioxidants and phytonutrients seem particularly helpful in retarding this terrible disease. Dietary recommendations include eating more carrots, spinach, collard greens, broccoli, apricots, blueberries, peppers, tomatoes, and pink grapefruit. Some of the most important nutrient supplements are listed below:

Highly Recommended:

Antioxidant supplements: Two per day
Beta-carotene: 25,000 IU per day
Vitamin E: 400 IU per day
Vitamin C: 1,000 mg per day
Lutein: 10–20 mg per day

Zinc: 50 mg per day
Bilberry: 80 mg three times per day
Taurine: 1,000–2,000 mg per day
Selenium: 200 mcg per day

Often Recommended:

Ginkgo biloba: 120–240 mg per day
Alpha-Lipoic acid: 100 mg per day
Grape seed extract: 100–200 mg per day

Menopausal Syndrome

The end of ovulation and cessation of menses characterize menopause. This natural phenomenon usually begins at approximately fifty-two years of age, although it can occur several years before or after. Women frequently complain of hot flashes, low libido, night sweats, mood swings, depression, vaginal dryness or itching, discomfort during intercourse, breast tenderness, palpitations, and insomnia. There is an increased risk of osteoporosis and heart disease after menopause.

While doctors all too frequently prescribe hormone replacement therapy involving synthetic estrogen and progesterone for women during menopause, proper diet, lifestyle changes, and nutritional supplements may alleviate many of the symptoms associated with menopause.

Many women have found that a combination of the vitamin B complex, additional vitamin B_6, calcium, magnesium, vitamin C with bioflavonoids, vitamin E, and herbal therapies such as black cohosh, dong quai, chasteberry, red clover, and ginseng may be helpful in alleviating menopausal hot flashes and depression. Essential fatty acids such as primrose oil or borage oil may also assist in reducing hot flashes.

There is also a type of natural hormone replacement therapy that your physician can prescribe and a compounding pharmacist can prepare. In this case, the quantity of estrogen and progesterone you take will be individualized to your specific needs. Furthermore, rather than taking a synthetic form of estrogen and progesterone that are structurally unnatural to what your body actually produces, these hormones are chemically identical to those you do produce in your body. I have been prescribing natural supplements and natural hormone replacement therapy to hundreds of women for more than fifteen years with excellent results. Many women report feeling more alive, energized, clear thinking, and that their depressions, hot flashes, insomnia, and nightly sweats have lifted.

Also effective in reducing menopausal symptoms is a high intake of soy products such as soybeans, tofu, and tempeh. It's also best to minimize dairy and red meat consumption because trace amounts of hormones, which may promote hot flashes, are frequently found in these foods. Particularly important is adequate intake of dark leafy vegetables, fresh fruit, beans, and whole grains. Regular weight-bearing exercise is another important adjunct.

When going through menopause, you may want to consider the following nutrients prior to initiating, or along with, synthetic hormone replacement therapy:

Highly Recommended:

Vitamin E: 400 IU three times per day
Vitamin C: 500 mg two times per day
Bioflavonoids: 500 mg two times per day
Black cohosh: 250 mg two times per day
Chasteberry (Vitex agnus cactus): 750 mg
two times per day
Dong quai: 500 mg two times per day
Soy isoflavones: 100 mg two times per day

Often Recommended:

Vitamin B$_6$: 50 mg two times per day
Vitamin B complex: 50 mg per day
Flaxseed oil: 1 tablespoon per day

Boron: 3 mg two times per day
Folic acid: 5 mg per day
Ginkgo biloba: 40 mg per day

Menorrhagia (Excessive menstrual bleeding)

Excessive menstrual bleeding, or menorrhagia, is an all-too-common problem that many women suffer from on a regular basis. It is essential that you consult with your physician to have him or her perform a thorough history and physical exam. If there are no obvious underlying causes, you might want to consider a nutritional approach, which can often help alleviate this condition:

Highly Recommended:

Vitamin C: 1,000 mg two times per day
Bioflavonoids: 1,000 mg two times per day

Vitamin A: 25,000 IU two times per day for two weeks followed by 25,000 IU per day thereafter
Iron: 100 mg per day

Often Recommended:

Vitamin E: 400 IU per day
Chlorophyll: 25 mg per day
Shepherd's purse: 250 mg two times per day

Chasteberry (Vitex agnus cactus): 40 drops of liquid extract per day or two 250 mg capsules per day

Health Tip: Shepherd's Purse

Shepherd's purse has been used to stop various forms of bleeding. It can be used as a tea or in capsule form to help women with hemorrhaging after childbirth. It can also be effective to reduce excessive menopausal bleeding. If drinking the tea, it is best to drink it cold.

Morning Sickness

Morning sickness frequently accompanies early pregnancy, especially in the first trimester. Although it is not thought of as a serious condition, it can still cause a significant amount of nausea and vomiting. Eating dry crackers upon arising and separating your liquids and solid foods may be mildly beneficial. You also might want to consider the following nutrients for relief:

Highly Recommended:

Vitamin K: 5 mg daily
Vitamin C: 500 mg two times per day
Vitamin B$_6$: 25 mg three times per day

Ginger: 25 mg two times per day, 1 cup of tea three times per day, or ½ teaspoon of tincture three times per day

Multiple Sclerosis

Multiple Sclerosis (MS) is a progressive degenerative neurologic disturbance caused by a gradual loss of the myelin sheath that surrounds nerve cells. If the myelin sheath is lost, neurologic function begins to deteriorate. MS more commonly arises between ages twenty and forty, and women are affected more frequently than men. There are numerous symptoms that can occur with MS, including weakness or stiffness in the legs, a tendency to drop things, clumsiness, a tingling sensation, numbness, blurred vision, double vision, lightheadedness, a sensation of feeling drunk, nausea, vomiting, loss of bladder control, and loss of sexual function.

There are numerous theories as to the cause of MS, ranging from an autoimmune process, viral infections, or even an excessive consumption of saturated animal fats and dairy products. A diet low in saturated fats and hydrogenated vegetable oils while high in cold-water fish such as salmon, cod, mackerel, and herring has been helpful for many people. Although it is highly controversial, there is some anecdotal evidence that demyelinization and MS can result from the accumulation of toxic metals such as mercury as found in "silver" dental fillings or certain types of fish. I use the following nutritional supplements with my MS patients:

Highly Recommended:

EPA/DHA fish oils: 2,000–4,000 mg per day

Flaxseed oil: 1 tablespoon per day

Multiple vitamin with minerals

Antioxidant formula: 2 capsules per day

Vitamin E: 800 IU per day

Selenium: 200 mcg two times per day

Pancreatic enzymes: 1,000–3,000 mg per day between meals

Calcium AEP: 3 capsules per day

Magnesium AEP: 3 capsules per day

Sphingomyelin: 2 capsules twice per day

Conjugated linoleic acid: 10 grams per day

Health Tip: Sphingomyelin

Sphingomyelin participates in the insulation around nerves that deteriorates in cases of MS. Although there is debate as to how absorbable the oral form might be, I nonetheless recommend an oral form of sphingomyelin known as Sphingolin (by Cardiovascular Research).

Health Tip: Conjugated Linoleic Acid

Supplements of linoleic acid (an omega-6 fatty acid) may help to reduce the disability, severity, and duration of relapses in people with MS. The benefits associated with linoleic acid are thought to be due to its effect on hormone-like substances known as prostaglandins.

Often Recommended:

Vitamin B_{12} (as methylcobalamin): 2–30 mg per day

Coenzyme Q_{10}: 100 mg two times per day

Phosphatidylserine: 100 mg two times per day

Ginkgo biloba: 60 mg three times per day

Obesity

Recent estimates indicate that nearly 50 percent of the adult population is now considered obese and close to one in every three children in the United States is overweight. Obesity can significantly increase your risk of dying prematurely from heart disease, cancer, stroke, or diabetes. As you know, there are numerous diets proposed for weight loss, some of which are very effective while others are virtually useless. It is my opinion that there is no one diet suitable for everyone since the metabolic needs, metabolism, and biochemistry differ from person to person. Similarly, there is not a magic bullet or quick fix for safe and permanent weight loss. A successful weight loss program entails reducing your caloric intake, consuming wholesome nutrient-dense unprocessed foods, getting adequate exercise, having a positive mental attitude, and using nutritional supplementation. Here are the nutrients which I have found helpful when combined with appropriate dietary and lifestyle modifications:

Highly Recommended:

Chromium: 400–600 mcg per day

Medium-chain triglycerides: 1–2 tablespoons per day

L-carnitine: 1,000–2,000 mg per day

5-Hydroxy L-tryptophan (5-HTP): 50–100 mg before meals

Hydroxycitric acid (HCA): 500 mg three times per day before meals

Coenzyme Q_{10}: 100 mg two times per day

Choline: 500 mg two times per day

Inositol: 500 mg two times per day

Health Tip: Medium-Chain Triglycerides

Medium-chain triglycerides are a type of fatty acid found in coconut oil and butter. They are more rapidly absorbed and burned as energy than long-chain fatty acids present in other fats and oils. It is best to consume these fatty acids with a meal to prevent gastrointestinal upset. Individuals with cirrhosis or other liver problems, however, should avoid them.

Health Tip: Hydroxycitric Acid (HCA)

Hydroxycitric acid (HCA) is a fruit extract derived from the rind of the Garcinia cambogia fruit, which is native to Southeast Asia. Preliminary research indicates that it may be useful for weight loss.

Often Recommended:

Conjugated linoleic acid: 1,000 mg two times per day

Fiber supplements: 8–10 grams per day

Osteoporosis

Osteoporosis is a disease in which the bones become progressively weaker as we age. This often leads to poor posture, shortened stature, and susceptibility to fractures. Nearly half of the female population in the United States over the age of forty-five show signs of early osteoporosis. The known risk factors for developing weak bones and progressive osteoporosis include cigarette smoking, a sedentary lifestyle, excessive alcohol, excessive caffeine, ingestion of aluminum-containing antacids, insufficient calcium intake, a high animal protein diet, and excessive sugar consumption. Light-skinned and small-framed individuals have also been shown to be at high risk.

Numerous nutritional factors play an important role in assisting new bone growth. Not only is calcium vitally important, but other key minerals such as magnesium, zinc, copper, manganese, silica, strontium, and boron are also essential. The lesser known naturally occurring substances glucosamine sulfate and chondroitin sulfate assist the body in manufacturing healthy bones and promoting the growth of new cartilage. Recent research indicates that vitamin K may also assist bone formation and calcium retention.

The following nutrients can be used both to prevent and treat osteoporosis:

Highly Recommended:

Calcium citrate or hydroxyapatite: 500 mg three times per day

Vitamin D: 400 IU per day

Boron: 3 mg two times per day

Magnesium: 400 mg two times per day

Vitamin K: 150 mcg two times per day

Silicon: 100 mg two times per day

Zinc: 15 mg per day

Soy isoflavones (ipriflavone): 200 mg three times per day

Multiple vitamin with minerals

Health Tip: Vitamin K

Vitamin K is needed not only for blood clotting but also for proper bone formation. I have found that many people with osteoporosis have low levels of vitamin K. In postmenopausal women with osteoporosis, vitamin K can help to reduce the excessive loss of calcium in the urine. Dietary sources of vitamin K include dark green leafy vegetables.

Health Tip: Silicon

Silicon is a trace mineral that is a vital component for the formation of bone and cartilage. The herb known as horsetail (in the form of *Equisetum arvense*) is particularly rich in silicon and may be beneficial in preventing osteoporosis in the form of a tea or ½–1 teaspoon of the tincture per day.

Often Recommended:

Folic acid: 1 mg per day

Chondroitin sulfate: 400 mg two times per day

Manganese: 10 mg per day

Glucosamine sulfate: 500 mg three times per day

Premenstrual Syndrome

Premenstrual syndrome (PMS) is usually characterized by one or a number of the following: irritability, tension, depression, mood swings, headaches, food cravings, breast tenderness, abdominal bloating, edema of the fingers or ankles, or fatigue that typically occurs seven to fourteen days before menstruation. Nutrition can play an important role in alleviating the symptoms. I strongly suggest that you reduce your intake of caffeine, sugar, salt, and saturated animal fats while trying to increase consumption of plant-based foods such as fresh fruit, vegetables, legumes, nuts, seeds, and whole grains. Eating more soy-based foods such as tofu, tempeh, soybeans, soy milk, and soy cheese and incorporating soy protein containing isoflavones is also helpful owing to their phytoestrogen content. I have also found the following nutrients very helpful in reducing symptoms of PMS:

Highly Recommended:

Vitamin B$_6$: 100 mg two times per day

Magnesium: 400 mg two times per day

Calcium: 500 mg two times per day

Vitamin E: 400 IU two times per day

Evening primrose oil: 1,300 mg two times per day

Dong quai fluid extract: ¼ teaspoon per day

Black cohosh: 250 mg two times per day

Chasteberry (Vitex agnus cactus): 200 mg per day

Vitamin B complex: 50 mg per day

Multiple vitamin with minerals

Often Recommended:

Zinc: 30 mg per day

Vitamin A: 25,000 IU per day

Prostate Enlargement

As men age, there is a gradual enlargement of the prostate gland, which sits just below the bladder and in front of the rectum. This condition is known as benign prostatic hyperplasia (BPH). It has been estimated that 50 percent of all men over the age of fifty and as many as 75 percent of those over seventy-five years old are affected. An enlarged prostate can lead to frequent urination, especially at night; reduction in urinary flow; and difficulty in starting or stopping urination. Physicians frequently prescribe medications as a man becomes more symptomatic. If drugs are unsuccessful, surgery may be necessary.

Natural approaches can be effective in reducing the size of the prostate gland. Herbs such as saw palmetto and *Pygeum africanum* have been used extensively for BPH in Europe and are now being more widely used in this country as well. In fact, they are often more effective than conventionally prescribed medications. There are also a wide range of other nutrients that may reduce prostate size, alleviate your symptoms, and lessen your need for medications.

If you are troubled with an enlarged prostate, the following may be helpful:

Highly Recommended:

Saw palmetto extract: 160 mg two times per day

Pygeum africanum extract: 50–100 mg two times per day

Stinging nettle: 120 mg two times per day

Zinc: 50 mg per day

Flaxseed oil: 1 tablespoon per day

Often Recommended:

Lycopene: 10 mg two times per day

Look for a product with a combination of the following amino acids: alanine, 200 mg per day; glutamic acid, 200 mg per day; and glycine, 200 mg per day

Pumpkin seed oil: 25 mg two times per day

Selenium: 200mcg per day

Health Tip: Lycopene

Lycopene is a carotenoid with potent antioxidant potential. It is commonly found in tomatoes and to a lesser degree in red grapefruit and watermelon. It appears that cooking tomatoes or tomato sauce can help to raise the lycopene level, thereby making it more bioavailable. Lycopene is an important substance to help prevent prostate cancer and cervical cancer, and to protect against vascular disease. Lycopene has also been found to protect LDL cholesterol from becoming oxidized, thereby lowering your risk for heart disease.

Psoriasis

Psoriasis is a common skin disorder where scaly, silvery plaques form on the skin, usually on the scalp, backs of the wrists, elbows, knees, back, ankles, trunk, and fingernails. Avoiding allergenic foods and alcohol can be beneficial at times. Improving your digestion, assimilation, liver function, and bowel function are also advisable. The following supplements are also of great benefit:

Highly Recommended:

Multiple vitamin with minerals
Flaxseed oil: 1 tablespoon per day
Fish oil capsules: 8,000–12,000 mg per day
Activated vitamin D (available by prescription): Apply topically two times per day

Zinc: 30 mg per day
Vitamin E: 400 IU per day
Vitamin A: 25,000 units one to two times per day

Health Tip: Activated Vitamin D

Activated vitamin D in the form of 1,25 dihydroxycholecalciferol can be applied topically in the treatment of psoriasis. It helps the skin cells replicate normally and is available by prescription from your dermatologist. Over-the-counter forms of oral vitamin D are of no significant benefit in the treatment of psoriasis.

Often Recommended:

Fumaric acid: 250 mg per day
Selenium: 200 mcg per day
Biotin: 1 mg two times per day
Silymarin: 100 mg three times per day
Psyllium husks: 5 mg two times per day
Goldenseal: 250 mg one–two times per day

Capsaicin topical cream: two times per day
Chamomile topical cream: two–three times per day

Health Tip: Fumaric Acid

Fumaric acid is more popular in Western Europe for the treatment of psoriasis than it is in the United States. Some studies indicate that it can be helpful in the treatment of psoriasis, but fumaric acid should only be used under the direction of a physician. Side effects can include nausea, diarrhea, general fatigue, gastric discomfort, or mild liver and kidney disturbances. For these reasons, use this therapy only after exhausting other, less troublesome treatments.

Health Tip: Capsaicin Topical Cream

Capsaicin is the active component found in cayenne pepper. This topical cream can help to reduce pain by depleting the neurotransmitter called substance P. Since substance P may stimulate inflammatory pathways in psoriasis, creams containing .025–.075 percent capsaicin may be effective in relieving psoriasis. I recommend washing your hands thoroughly after its use or to wear gloves when applying capsaicin cream. Be careful not to touch your eyes, nose, mouth, or other mucous membranes since it can cause a burning sensation.

Health Tip: Chamomile Topical Cream

Chamomile topical cream contains anti-inflammatory and anti-allergy properties and has been used to treat a variety of skin disorders including psoriasis, eczema, and irritated skin.

Rosacea

Rosacea is a chronic skin condition typically affecting the nose and cheeks of adults between the ages of thirty and fifty. Women are affected three times more frequently than men. Symptoms can include redness, acne-like eruptions, facial swelling, or dilated capillaries. Avoid allergenic foods, and make sure your gastrointestinal tract secretes optimal amounts of pancreatic enzymes and hydrochloric acid. I also recommend that you try to avoid alcohol, caffeine, hot beverages, spicy foods, simple sugars, milk, and trans-fatty acids, which are found in fried foods and hydrogenated vegetable oils. Supplements can give some relief from symptoms of rosacea:

Highly Recommended:

Betaine hydrochloride (HCL): Dose needs to be determined by a nutritionally oriented physician. Most people start with 5–10 grain (325–650 mg) tablets or capsules along with a meal that contains protein. If intestinal burning occurs, HCL should be discontinued immediately.

Pancreatin: 500 mg before meals
Vitamin B complex: 50 mg per day
Multiple vitamin with minerals

Health Tip: Betaine Hydrochloride

Betaine hydrochloride is a form of hydrochloric acid that is naturally produced by the parietal cells of the stomach in response to the ingestion of food. This substance assists in the absorption of vitamins and minerals and other nutrients. Unfortunately, with advancing age, hydrochloric acid production frequently declines. Supplements should not be taken along with aspirin-containing compounds or other anti-inflammatory drugs including steroids. Excessive amounts of betaine hydrochloride can cause gastric irritation or bleeding if combined with these medications.

Sinus Infections

Sinus infections occur when the mucous membranes swell and drainage from the sinuses is blocked. Bacteria can then multiply, leading to infection. The common cold, an upper respiratory infection, a dental infection, or immune weakness that causes hay fever or food allergies are all-important factors that can predispose you to sinusitis. Typically, you might feel pain or pressure around the eyes or nose or perhaps develop a yellow-green mucus discharge. Although doctors frequently prescribe antibiotics to treat acute sinus infections, I have found that improving your immune response, removing inhalant and food allergies, avoiding chemical exposures to, for example, new carpeting or cleaning detergents, are helpful approaches. Many of my patients respond favorably to the avoidance of milk, wheat, and sugar as well as flushing the nasal passages with a solution of salt and warm water. I limit the use of antibiotics to treat sinus infections since they might encourage an overgrowth of yeast in the body. There are a variety of nutritional supplements that may be just as effective as antibiotics, and these are listed below:

Highly Recommended:

Vitamin C: 1,000 mg three times per day

Bioflavonoids: 1,000 mg two times per day

Vitamin A: 25,000 IU per day

Bromelain: 500 mg two times per day between meals

Echinacea: 250 mg capsule or ½–1 teaspoon of the extract two times per day

Goldenseal: 250 mg two times per day

Often Recommended:

Beta-carotene: 25,000 IU per day

Zinc: 30 mg per day

Maitake D-fraction: 30 drops per day

Beneficial bacteria such as *lactobacillus* and *bifidobacterium*: 1–3 billion organisms per day

Sore Throat

All of us have probably suffered a sore throat at some time during our life. Sore throats are typically caused by viruses although they can be caused by a bacteria known as Group A beta hemolytic streptococci. Sore throat symptoms typically include pain on swallowing, tender lymph nodes, swollen tonsils, and a red throat. If you have been on numerous antibiotics in the past, I suggest supplementing with a probiotic that contains *lactobacillus acidophilus* and *bifidobacterium*. It is also important to change your toothbrush on a regular basis. The following are some of the nutrients that can help accelerate healing and reduce your sore throat symptoms:

Highly Recommended:

Vitamin C: 1,000 mg three times per day

Bioflavonoids: 1,000 mg three times per day

Vitamin A: 25,000 IU two times per day for one week

Zinc throat lozenges: 1 every three hours

Echinacea: 500 mg capsule or ½–1 teaspoon of the fluid extract three times per day

Goldenseal: 250 mg two times per day

Often Recommended:

Beta-carotene: 25,000 IU three times per day

Ginger tea: 1 cup two times per day

Ulcers

Both stomach and intestinal ulcers can cause abdominal tenderness, pain, heartburn, or rectal bleeding. For many years, ulcers were thought to be a result of stress. However, a bacteria known as *Helicobacter pylori* may be a predisposing factor in developing an ulcer. It has also been well documented that taking aspirin or nonsteroidal anti-inflammatory agents on a regular basis can also increase your risk of developing an ulcer. If you have been diagnosed with an ulcer, there are several natural therapies that you should consider.

Highly Recommended:

High-fiber diet
Raw cabbage juice: 4 oz per day
Glutamine: 500–1,000 mg three times per day
Buffered vitamin C: 500 mg three times per day

Vitamin A: 10,000 IU per day
Zinc: 30 mg per day
Bioflavonoids: 500 mg three times per day
Deglycyrrhizinated licorice (DGL): 2–4 380 mg chewable tablets three times per day before meals

Health Tip: Glutamine

Glutamine, an amino acid, is one of the major sources of fuel for cells lining the intestinal tract and stomach. I have found glutamine to be helpful in accelerating healing for peptic ulcers.

Health Tip: Deglycyrrhizinated Licorice (DGL)

DGL is very effective in treating peptic ulcer disease. In this form, the portion of the licorice root associated with high blood pressure and fluid retention in some people has been removed, making DGL a very safe product. DGL has also been helpful in soothing inflamed and irritated mucous membranes of the gastrointestinal tract.

Often Recommended:

Vitamin E: 400 IU per day
Quercetin: 500 mg three times per day

Chamomile tea: 2–3 cups or 1 teaspoon of the tincture in warm water per day

Varicose Veins

Varicose veins, which occur when the superficial veins of the legs grow tortuous or dilated, affects nearly 50 percent of the middle-aged population. Varicose veins occur more frequently in women (especially after pregnancy), in obese individuals, and in people who are standing for long periods of time. Although they are not truly hazardous to your health, most people find varicose veins cosmetically unpleasing.

Eating a high-complex-carbohydrate, high-fiber diet while avoiding a low-fiber, highly refined diet is important here. Keeping your bowels moving on a regular basis and drinking at least six glasses of water per day can also be helpful. Getting regular exercise can promote contraction of the leg muscles to reduce the pooling of blood in the varicose veins. Nutritional supplements are quite helpful including the following:

Highly Recommended:

Horse chestnut: 250 mg two times per day
Grape seed extract or Pycnogenol®: 150 mg two times per day
Butcher's broom: 100 mg three times per day

Vitamin C: 1,000 mg three times per day
Vitamin E: 400 IU per day
Bioflavonoids: 500 mg two times per day

Often Recommended:

Bromelain: 500 mg three times per day between meals

Bilberry: 80 mg three times per day
Zinc: 30 mg per day

Yeast Infections

Yeast infections are a common problem that cause women to seek treatment. Symptoms can include irritation, inflammation, discomfort on urination, or a complaint of a vaginal discharge. Vaginal yeast infections, which are typically caused by the fungal organism *Candida albicans*, is more prevalent in women who have taken oral antibiotics, birth control pills, steroids, or are eating a high-sugar diet. If you have noticed a thick, curdy, or "cottage cheese" discharge, you should consult with a health-care professional to confirm the diagnosis of yeast. Although there are several prescription and over-the-counter medications to help treat this condition, the following natural therapies may also be helpful:

Highly Recommended:

Beneficial bacteria: 1–3 billion live organisms per day

Multiple vitamin with minerals

Caprylic acid: 2–4 capsules per day

Oil of oregano: 2–4 drops per day

Vitamin C: 1,000 mg three times per day

Garlic capsules: 500 mg three times per day

Often Recommended:

Goldenseal: 250 mg capsule three times per day

Echinacea: 250 mg teaspoon (1) per day

Pau D'Arco: 30 drops three times per day

Tea tree oil douche: Mix 1 teaspoon of a 20% solution per pint of warm water

Boric acid capsules: 600 mg vaginal suppository two times per day (available by prescription from compounding pharmacy)

REFERENCES AND SUGGESTED FURTHER READING

Part I

Adderly, Brenda D., M.H.A. *The Complete Guide to Nutritional Supplements: Everything You Need to Make Informed Choices for Optimum Health*, New Star Press, 1998.

Atkins, Robert, M.D. *Dr. Atkins' New Diet Revolution*, M. Evans and Company, Inc., 1999.

Atkins, Robert, M.D. *Dr. Atkins' Vita-Nutrient Solution*, Simon & Schuster, 1998.

Atlas, Nava. *Whole Food Catalog: A Complete Guide to Natural Food*, Fawcett Columbine Publishers, 1988.

Balch, James E., M.D., and Balch, Phyllis A., C.N.C. *Prescription for Nutritional Healing*, Avery Publishing Group, 1997.

Carper, Jean. *Stop Aging Now*, HarperCollins Publications, 1995.

Cooper, Kenneth, M.D. *Kenneth Cooper's Antioxidant Revolution*, Thomas Nelson Publishers, 1994.

Crook, William G., M.D. *The Yeast Connection Handbook,* Professional Books, 1996.

Gaynor, Mitchell, M.D., and Hickey, Jerry, R.Ph. *Dr. Gaynor's Cancer Prevention Program,* Kensington Books, 1999.

Golan, Ralph, M.D. *Optimal Wellness*, Random House, 1995.

Griffith, H. Winter, M.D. *Vitamins, Herbs, Minerals & Supplements. The Complete Guide*. Fisher Books, 1998.

Haas, Elson, M.D. *Staying Healthy with Nutrition*, Celestial Arts, 1992.

Janson, Michael, M.D. *The Vitamin Revolution in Health Care*, Arcadia Press, 1996.

Kalyn, Wayne, Ed. *The Healing Power of Vitamins, Minerals and Herbs,* Reader's Digest Association, 1999.

Kirschmann, Gayla J., and Kirschmann, John D. *Nutrition Almanac,* Fourth Edition, McGraw-Hill, 1996.

Lieberman, Shari, Ph.D., and Brunnig, Nancy. *The Real Vitamin and Mineral Book,* Avery Publishing Group, 1997.

Magaziner, Allan, D.O. *The Complete Idiot's Guide to Living Longer and Healthier,* Alpha Books, 1999.

Murray, Michael T., N.D. *Encyclopedia of Nutritional Supplements,* Prima Publishing, 1996.

Ornish, Dean, M.D. *Dr. Dean Ornish's Program for Reversing Heart Disease,* Random House, 1990.

Pirello, Christina. *Cooking the Whole Foods Way*, HP Books, 1997.

Pressman, Alan H., D.C., Ph.D., with Buff, Sheila. *The GSH Phenomenon*, St. Martin's Press, 1997.

Rapp, Doris, M.D. *Is This Your Child?* William Morrow & Company, Inc., 1991.

Remington, Dennis W., M.D., and Higa, Barbara W., R.D. *The Bitter Truth About Artificial Sweeteners,* Vitality House International, 1987.

Robbins, John. *Diet for a New America,* Stilllpoint Publishing, 1987.

Simopoulos, Artemis P., M.D., and Robinson, Jo. *The Omega Plan,* HarperCollins, 1998.

Sinatra, Stephen T., M.D. *The CoEnzyme Q_{10} Phenomenon,* Keats Publishing, 1998.

Somer, Elizabeth, M.A., R.D. *Food and Mood: The Complete Guide to Eating Well and Feeling Your Best,* 1995.

U.S. Department of Health and Human Services, National Institute of Health, NIH Publication No. 93-2922 "So You Have High Blood Cholesterol," 1993.

Wright, Jonathan V., M.D. *Dr. Wright's Guide to Healing with Nutrition,* Keats Publishing, Inc. 1990.

Part II

Braly, James, M.D. *Dr. Braly's Food Allergy and Nutrition Revolution,* Keats Publishing, Inc., 1992.

Krohn, Jacqueline, M.D. *The Whole Way to Allergy Relief & Prevention,* Hartley & Marks Publishers, 1996.

Null, Gary, Ph.D. *No More Allergies,* Villard Books, 1992.

Rapp, Doris, M.D. *Is This Your Child?* William Morrow & Company, Inc., 1991.

Rapp, Doris, M.D. *Is This Your Child's World?* Bantam Books, 1996.

Rea, William, M.D. *Chemical Sensitivity,* Volumes I and II, Lewis Publishers, 1992.

Rea, William, M.D. and Golos, Natalie. *Success in the Clean Bedroom,* Pinnacle Publishers, 1992.

Part III

Bower, Lynn Marie. *The Healthy Household,* The Healthy Household Institute, 1995.

Dickey, Lawrence D., M.D., Ed. *Clinical Ecology,* Charles C Thomas Publisher, 1976.

Fincher, Cynthia E., Ph.D. *Healthy Living in a Toxic World,* Pinon Press, 1996.

Gorman, Carolyn P., B.A., M.A. *Less Toxic Living,* Environmental Health Center, 1993.

Krohn, Jacqueline, M.D. *The Whole Way to Allergy Relief & Prevention,* Hartley & Marks Publishers, 1996.

Rapp, Doris, M.D. *Is This Your Child's World?* Bantam Books, 1996.

Rea, William, M.D. *Chemical Sensitivities,* Volumes I and II, Lewis Publishers, 1992.

Rea, William, M.D. and Golos, Natalie. *Success in the Clean Bedroom,* Pinnacle Publishers, 1992.

Part IV

Burton Goldberg Group, *Alternative Medicine: The Definitive Guide,* Future Medicine Publishing, Inc., 1999.

Chopra, Deepak, M.D. *Perfect Health: The Complete Mind/Body Guide,* Harmony Books, 1991.

Chopra, Deepak, M.D. *The Seven Spiritual Laws of Success*, Amber-Allen Publishing, 1994.

Golan, Ralph, M.D. *Optimal Wellness*, Ballantine Books, 1995.

Larson, Joan Mathews, Ph.D. *Seven Weeks to Sobriety*, Fawcett Columbine, 1997.

Magaziner, Allan, D.O. *The Complete Idiot's Guide to Living Longer and Healthier*, Alpha Books, 1999.

Myss, Caroline, Ph.D. *Why People Don't Heal and How They Can*, Three Rivers Press, 1997.

Weil, Andrew, M.D. *Spontaneous Healing*, Ballantine Books, 1995.

Part V

Barney, Paul, M.D. *Doctor's Guide to Natural Medicine*, Woodland Publishing, 1998.

Bland, Jeffrey, Ph.D. *The 20-Day Rejuvenation Diet Program*, Keats Publishing, 1997.

Brecher, Arline, and Brecher, Harold. *Forty-Something Forever*, Health Savers Press, 1998.

Burton Goldberg Group, *Alternative Medicine: The Definitive Guide*, Future Medicine Publishing, Inc., 1999.

Burton Goldberg Group. *Alternative Medicine Guide to Heart Disease*, Future Medicine Publishing, Inc., 1998.

Chappell, Terry, M.D. *Questions from the Heart*, Hampton Roads Publishing Company, Inc., 1995.

Cranton, Elmer, M.D. *Bypassing Bypass: The New Technique of Chelation Therapy*, Hampton Roads Publishing Company, Inc., 1992.

Diamond, W. John, M.D., and Cowden, W. Lee, M.D. *An Alternative Medicine Definitive Guide to Cancer*, Future Medicine Publishing, Inc., 1997.

Epstein, Samuel, M.D., and Steinman, David. *The Breast Cancer Prevention Program*, Macmillan Publishing, 1997.

Gaby, Alan, M.D., *Preventing and Reversing Osteoporosis*, Prima Publishing, 1994.

Jonas, Wayne B., M.D., and Jacobs, Jennifer, M.D., M.P.H. *Healing with Homeopathy,* Warner Books, 1996.

Lininger, Skye, D.C., Ed. *The Natural Pharmacy*, Prima Publishing, 1998.

Lockie, Andrew, M.D., and Geddes, Nicola, M.D. *The Complete Guide to Homeopathy: The Principles and Practice of Treatment,* DK Publishing, Inc., 1995.

Lombard, Jay, D.O., and Germano, Carl, R.D. *The Brain Wellness Plan*, Kensington Books, 1997.

McCully, Kilmer, M.D. *The Heart Revolution*, HarperCollins, 1999.

Magaziner, Allan, D.O. *The Complete Idiot's Guide to Living Longer and Healthier*, Alpha Books, 1999.

Mindell, Earl, R.Ph., Ph.D. *Earl Mindell's Secret Remedies*, Simon & Schuster, 1997.

Murray, Michael T., N.D. *The Healing Power of Herbs*, Prima Publishing, 1995.

Murray, Michael T., N.D., and Pizzorno, Joseph, N.D. *Encyclopedia of Natural Medicine*, Prima Publishing, 1998.

Northrup, Christiane, M.D. *Women's Bodies, Women's Wisdom*, Bantam Books, 1998.

Null, Gary, Ph.D. *The Clinician's Handbook of Natural Healing*, Kensington Books, 1997.

Null, Gary, Ph.D. *The Complete Encyclopedia of Natural Healing*, Kensington Books, 1998.

Null, Gary, Ph.D. *Gary Null's Ultimate Anti-Aging Program*, Kensington Books, 1999.

Peirce, Andrea. *Practical Guide to Natural Medicines*, William Morrow and Company, 1999.

Pizzorno, Joseph, N.D. *Total Wellness*, Prima Publishing, 1996.

Quillin, Patrick, Ph.D., R.D., C.N.S. *Beating Cancer with Nutrition*, Nutrition Times Press, Inc., 1998.

Rodale Press, *Natural Prescriptions for Women*, 1998.

Rose, Barry, *The Family Health Guide to Homeopathy*, Celestial Arts, 1992.

Santillo, Humbart, N.D. *Natural Healing with Herbs*, Hohm Press, 1993.

Sinatra, Stephen T., M.D. *Heartbreak and Heart Disease*, Keats Publishing, Inc., 1996.

Sinatra, Stephen T., M.D. *Optimum Health: A Natural Lifesaving Prescription for Your Body and Mind*, Bantam Books, 1997.

Somer, Elizabeth, M.A., R.D. *Age-Proof Your Body,* William Morrow and Company, Inc., 1998.

Theodosakis, Jason, M.D., Adderly, Brenda, M.H.A., and Fox, Barry, Ph.D. *The Arthritis Cure*, St. Martin's Press, 1997.

Ullman, Robert, N.D., and Reichenberg-Ullman, Judyth, N.D. *Homeopathic Self Care*, Prima Publishing, 1997.

Walker, Morton, D.P.M., and Shah, Hitendra, M.D. *Everything You Should Know About Chelation Therapy*, Keats Publishing, 1997.

Werbach, Melvyn, M.D. *Nutritional Influence on Illness*, Second Edition, Third Line Press, 1996.

Whitaker, Julian, M.D. *Reversing Diabetes*, Warner Books, 1987.

ADDENDUM

From Lane Labs. See Appendix I: Resource Guide for contact information.

I'm always searching for the latest information and products to help my patients achieve and maintain optimum health. This book contains many of them. However, after I completed the book, I learned of a new, natural immune stimulator called MGN-3. In using it with a number of patients, I found MGN-3 to be highly effective in enhancing Natural Killer cells, B-cells and T-cells—the immune system's first line of defense. Extensive human clinical research involving patients with HIV and cancer has been conducted using MGN-3, with dramatic results.

APPENDIX I

Resource Guide

I am frequently asked which brand of vitamins and other nutritional supplements I commonly recommend. There are certainly a wide range of products on the market and hundreds of manufacturers today. Select companies that have a long history of quality products, a proven track record, a reputation for good quality control, and reasonable prices. Over the years I have recommended hundreds of products from several different manufacturers. The following list is a list of brand names of nutritional supplements that you may want to select. They are usually available in your local health food store.

The following is a list of companies and their phone numbers for consumer information. These companies have multi products within this resource section. Those companies with a singular product or line will have their contact information listed within the context of the resource section.

Dr. Magaziner's Top Nutritional Supplement Companies

Allergy Research Group
30806 Santana Street
Hayward, CA 94544
1-800-545-9960
510-487-8526

Biometrics, Inc. (1-800-724-5566)

Carlson® Laboratories
15 College Drive
Arlington Heights, IL 60004-1985
1-888-234-5656
847-255-1600

Healthy Impact, Inc.
Davie, FL 33317 (888-523-3111)

Jarrow Formulas, Inc.™
1824 South Robertson Blvd.
Los Angeles, CA 90035-4317
1-800-726-0886
310-204-6936

Lane Labs
110 Commerce Drive
Allendale, NJ 07401
800-526-3005
201-236-9090 (Int'l)

Natrol®
21411 Prairie St.
Chatsworth, CA 91311
1-800-326-1520
818-739-6000
http://www.natrol.com

Nature's Plus
548 Broadhollow Road
Melville, NY 11747 (1-800-937-0500)

NutriCology (subsidiary of Scottsdale Scientific, Inc.)
419 Mission Street
San Rafael, CA 94901 (888-563-1506)

Prevail Corporation
2204 NW Birdsdale
Gresham, OR 97030
1-800-248-0885
503-667-4790
www.prevail.com

Planetary Formulas
23 Janis Way
Scotts Valley, CA 95066 (408-438-1144)

Solgar Vitamin & Herb
500 Willow Tree Road
Leonia, NJ 07605 (1-800-645-2246)

Source Naturals®
23 Janis Way
Scotts Valley, CA 96066 (408-438-1144)
http://www.sourcenaturals.com
    Products available at fine healthfood stores everywhere.

Wakunaga of America
23501 Madero
Mission Viejo, CA 92691 (1-800-421-2998)

Vitamin A

Available from the following companies:

Carlson®
PRODUCT NAME: Vitamins A & D
CONTAINS: Vitamin A, from fish liver oil, 10,000 i.u. and Vitamin D_3, from fish liver oil, 400 i.u.
Available in softgels

Source Naturals ™
PRODUCT NAME: Vitamin A
CONTAINS: 10,000 i.u. in tablet form

Allergy Control

Available from the following company:

Prevail
PRODUCT NAME: Sinease ™
CONTAINS: Bioflavonoids, Eyebright, Ephedra Extract
Available in capsules

Acid Indigestion/Heartburn

Available from the following company:

Prevail
PRODUCT NAMES: Acid-Ease®
CONTAINS: Pure Plant Enzymes, Slippery Elm, Marshmallow Root.
Available in capsules

Acidophilus

Available from the following company:

Prevail
PRODUCT NAME: Inner Ecology®
CONTAINS: L. acidophilus and other microflora with FOS
Available in powder

Alpha Lipoic Acid

Available form the following companies:

Allergy Research Group
PRODUCT NAME: ThioDox™
CONTAINS: N-Acetyl-Cysteine, Glutathione, Lipoic Acid, TTFD, Riboflavin 5 Phosphate, Asorbic Acid, and L-Selenomethionine. Available in tablets.
Carlson®
PRODUCT NAME: Alpha Lipoic Acid
Available in 100mg tablets

Jarrow Formulas™
PRODUCT NAME: Alpha Liopic Sustain 300
Sustained released tablets, 300mg each

Source Naturals™
PRODUCT NAME: Lipoic Acid
Available in 200mg tablets

Amino Acids

Available from the following company:

Allergy Research Group
PRODUCT NAME: Free Aminos™
CONTAINS: 17 naturally occurring amino acids in their free forms, including 9 essential amino acids. Does not contain tryptophan. Available in capsules or powder.

Antitoxidants

Available from the following companies:

Carlson®
PRODUCT NAME: Aces Gold™
CONTAINS: Vitamin E, Zinc, Selenium, Co-Q10, Glutathione, N-Acetyl Cysteine, Alpha Lipoic, Citrus Bioflavonoids, Quercetin, Garlic, Grape Seed Extract, Green Tea, and others.
RECOMMENDED: 2 tablets daily at mealtime

Natrol®
PRODUCT NAME: The Ultimate Anti-Oxidant Formula
CONTAINS: Vitamins A, C, and E, Niacinamide, Copper, and Zinc
Available in capsules

Source Naturals
PRODUCT NAME: Super Beta Carotene
CONTAINS: 20,000 i.u. in softgel form

Prevail
PRODUCT NAME: Plant Source® Antioxidants
CONTAINS: Beta Carotene, Vitamin C and E, Zinc, Grape Seed Extract, Pine Bark, Lycopenes
Available in Capsules

Astragalus/Echinacea

Available from the following company:

Prevail
PRODUCT NAME: Defense Formula
CONTAINS: Astragalus, Echinacea, Vitamin C, Shiitake
Available in capsules

PRODUCT NAME: Defense Throat Lozenge
CONTAINS: Astragalus, Echinacea, Zinc, Licorice Root
Available in lozenge tablet

B-Complex (contains all of the individual B Vitamins)

Available from the following companies:

Carlson®
PRODUCT NAME: B-50 Gel
Balanced B-Complex in softgel form

PRODUCT NAME: Time-B®
Timed-Release: 50mg tablets

Jarrow Formulas™
PRODUCT NAME: B-Right™
Balanced B-Complex in capsule form

Source Naturals
PRODUCT NAME: CoEnzymate™ B Complex
Sublingual (dissolves under the tongue and goes directly into bloodstream) tablets in pep-
    permint and orange flavors with CO-Q10

B12

Available from the following company:

Source Naturals
PRODUCT NAME: B-12
Dibencozide Sublingual CoEnzymanted ™ B-12

Beta Carotene

Available from the following companies:

Jarrow Formulas™
PRODUCT NAME: Marine Beta Carotene™
Available in 15mg softgels

Source Naturals®
PRODUCT NAME: Beta Carotene
Pro-Vitamin A
CONTAINS: 20,000 i.u. Vitamin A in softgel form

PRODUCT NAME: SuperBeta Carotene™
All-natural, derived from single-cell algae, available in softgel form

Bilberry (contains active ingredients which affect proper eye function)

Available from the following companies:

Carlson®
PRODUCT NAME: Bilberry
CONTAINS: Potent Standardized Bilberry plus Vitamins A and E
In 25mg softgels

Jarrow Formulas™
PRODUCT NAME: Bilberry 100:1 and Grapeskin Polyphenols
Available in 280 mg capsules

Natrol®
PRODUCT NAME: Bilberry 25%
CONTAINS: 100:1 Bilberry Extract in capsule form

Solgar
PRODUCT NAME: Bilberry
Available in 260mg Vegicaps®

Source Naturals™
PRODUCT NAME: Bilberry Extract
Standardized to 25% Anthocyanosides
Available in 100mg tablets

Black Cohosh

Available from the following companies:

Prevail
PRODUCT NAME: Meno-Fem®
CONTAINS: Black Cohosh, Wild Yam, Dong Quai
Available in capsules

Source Naturals®
PRODUCT NAME: Hot Flash
CONTAINS: 160 mg Black Cohosh, 2,500 mg Soy-Life TM Genistein-Rich soy concentrate, 150 mg Dong Quai Extract, 150 mg Licorice Root Extract, 100 mg Vitex Extract

Borage (oil)

Available from the following company:

Jarrow Formulas™
PRODUCT NAME: Borage GLA-240 and Ganna Tocopherol
240mg Gammalinolenic Acid (GLA) in softgel form

Vitamin C and Ester C©

Available from the following companies:

Jarrow Formulas™
PRODUCT NAME: Vitamin C 1000
CONTAINS: 1000mg Vitamin C and 50mg Rosemary in capsule form

Natrol®
PRODUCT NAME: ESTER-C® 500 mg with Bioflavonoids
Available in 500mg capsules and tablets

Calcium

Available form the following company:

Source Naturals®
PRODUCT NAME: ULTRA-CAL NIGHT (Krebs Cycle Calcium Complex)
CONTAINS: 600 mg Calcium (Citrate, Malate, Fumerate, Ethanolamine Phosphate and Ascorbate); 600 mg of Magnesium (Oxide, Citrate, Fumerate, Malate and Ascorbates) as well as nutrients.

Cod Liver Oil

Available from the following company:

Carlson®
PRODUCT NAME: Norwegian Cod Liver Oil
CONTAINS: 500-550mg DHA, 460-500mg EPA, and 46-50mg ALA
In liquid form

Co-Q10

Available from the following companies:

Jarrow Formulas™
PRODUCT NAME: Co-Q10
Coenzyme Q-10, Pharmaceutical Grade, available in 30mg, 60mg, and 100mg capsules
For maximum absorption, also available in proliposome format in 30mg softgels

Solgar
PRODUCT NAME: Coenzyme Q-10
Available in 30mg and 100mg softgels

Source Naturals®
PRODUCT NAME: Coenzyme Q10 with Bioperine®
Available in 30mg softgels

PRODUCT NAME: Coenzyme Q10 Lipoic Acid
Available in 30mg capsules

PRODUCT NAME: Ultra Potency Coenzyme Q10
Available in 125mg capsules

Cranberry

Available from the following company:

Prevail
PRODUCT NAME: Urinary Tract EnzymeFormula
CONTAINS: Cranberry, Dandelion, Goldenrod, Horsetail and Astragalus
Available in capsules

Detoxification

Available from the following company:

Prevail
PRODUCT NAME: Detox Enzyme Formula® supports the liver and detoxification pathways
CONTAINS: Vitamin A, C and E, N-Acetyl-L-Cysteine, amino acids
Available in capsules

PRODUCT NAME: Metabolic Liver Formula supports the liver in processing nutrients, hormones and toxins
CONTAINS: Contains Mile Thistle, choline, methionine, inositol, Black Radish Root, and Beet Leaf
Available in capsules

DHA (necessary for tissue building in the brain and retina)

Available from the following companies:

Allergy Research Group
PRODUCT NAME: DHA—Fish Oil Concentrate
Available in 330mg softgels

Carlson®
PRODUCT NAME: Super DHA™, from fish oil
Available in 500mg softgels

Jarrow Formulas™
PRODUCT NAME: Max DHA™, 50 % DHA, 20 % EPA
Available in 505mg softgels

Martek
Supplier of Neuromins® DHA, a special micro-algae, non-fish DHA product in softgel form. For information and a list of companies carrying Neuromins®, call 1-800-662-6339.

Digestive Enzymes

Available from the following companies:

Jarrow Formulas™
PRODUCT NAME: Jarrow-Zymes™ Plus
Cold-extracted Pancreatin with Lipase and Alpha Galactosidase
Available in 425mg capsules

Natrol®
PRODUCT NAME: Digest Support™
CONTAINS: Proteolytic Enzymes, Amylolytic Enzymes, Lipolytic Enzymes, and Anti Gas Factor
Available in capsules

Prevail
PRODUCT NAME: Vitase® Digestion Formula
CONTAINS: Pure Plant Enzymes
Available in capsule

PRODUCT NAME: Bean & Vegi Enzyme Formula
CONTAINS: Pure Plant Enzymes
Available in capsules

PRODUCT NAME: Children's Vitase R Digestion Formula
CONTAINS: Pure Plant Enzymes
Available in capsules

Source Naturals®
PRODUCT NAME: Essential Enzymes™
CONTAINS: 500 mg of full-spectrum enzymatic activity. All vegetarian, high potency, broad-spectrum blend of lipase, amylase and protease. Available in 500 mg capsules.

Vitamin E

Available from the following companies:

Carlson®
PRODUCT NAME: E-Gems®
Available in 30-1200 i.u. softgels

PRODUCT NAME: E-Sel
CONTAINS: Vitamin E 400 I.U.
Available in softgels

Natrol®
PRODUCT NAME: Vitamin E 400 I.U.
Available in softgels

Echinacea

Available from the following companies:

Carlson®
PRODUCT NAME: Echinacea plus Vitamin C
CONTAINS: 100mg Echinacea Extract and 250mg Vitamin C
In softgel form

Jarrow Formulas®
PRODUCT NAME: Echinacea Super 3
Made with super concentrates, available in 226mg capsules

Eye Formulations

Carlson®
PRODUCT NAME: Eye-Rite™
CONTAINS: Lutein, Bilberry Extract, Cranberry Extract, Grape Seed Extract, Citrus Bio-flavonoid Complex, Quercetin, Soy Isoflavone Concentrate, Alpha Lipoic, Vitamin E, Vitamin C, Vitamin A, Zinc, Chromium, and Spirulina-Algae. In capsule form.

Natrol®
PRODUCT NAME: Eye Support w/Bilberry
CONTAINS: Bilberry Fruit Extract, Blueberry Leaf, Eyebright Leaf, Rasberry Leaf, Barberry Leaf, and Pulsatilla Leaf. In capsule form.

NutriCology®
PRODUCT NAME: OcuDyne II with Lutein
CONTAINS: NAC, Bilberry Extract, Ginkgo Biloba, Quercetin, Taurine, L-Methionine, Silicon, Lutein, and important minerals and B Vitamins. In capsule form.

Planetary Formula (Michael Tierra, C.A., N.D.)
PRODUCT NAME: Bilberry Eye Complex
Available in 643mg tablets

PRODUCT NAME: Bilberry Vision
CONTAINS: Bilberry Extract, yielding 37% Anthocyanosides
Available in 100mg tablets

Source Naturals
PRODUCT NAME: Visual-Eyes
Multi-Nutrient Complex
CONTAINS: Bilberry Extract, Lipoic Acid, Lutein, Ginkgo Bilboa, Quercetin, NAC, Taurine, and Inositol. Includes other synergistic vitamins and minerals.
Available in tablet form.

Fish Oil

Available from the following company:

Prevail
PRODUCT NAME: Eskimo-3®
Natural stable fish oil with Vitamin E. Contains omega-3, EPA and DHA.
Available in soft gel capsules

Flaxseed Oil

Available from the following companies:

Jarrow Formulas™
PRODUCT NAME: Flaxseed Oil™
Certified organic vegetarian omega-3, available in 1000mg capsules

Source Naturals®
PRODUCT NAME: Flax Seed-Primrose Oil
ALA and GLA complex
Available in 1300mg softgels

Folic Acid

Available from the following company:

Jarrow Formulas™
PRODUCT NAME: Folic Acid
Available in 800mg capsules

Garlic

Available from the following companies:

Carlson®
PRODUCT NAME: Garlic-600
Odorless garlic supplement, available in 600mg tablets

Wakunaga of America
PRODUCT NAME: KyolicR Aged Garlic Extract™
Organically grown, 100% odorless

Ginger

Available from the following company:

Jarrow Formulas™
PRODUCT NAME: Freeze Dried Ginger
6:1 Concentrate, available in 500mg capsules

Ginkgo Biloba

Available from the following companies:

Carlson®
PRODUCT NAME: Ginkgo Biloba plus L-Glutamine
CONTAINS: 40mg Ginkgo Biloba Extract and 200mg L-Glutamine
In softgel form

Jarrow Formulas™
PRODUCT NAME: Ginkgo Biloba 50:1
Available in 40mg and 60mg capsules and tablets

Prevail
PRODUCT NAME: Maxi-Mind
CONTAINS: Ginkgo biloba (24%), DMAE, Gotu Kola and Brahmi
Available in capsules

Glucosamine Sulfate

Available from the following companies:

Jarrow Formulas™
PRODUCT NAME: Glucosamine Sulfate 500
Sodium free, available in 670mg capsules

Prevail
PRODUCT NAME: Mobil-Ease
CONTAINS: Glucosamine sulfate 500 mg, Boswellia and White Willow Bark
Available in capsules

Glutathione

Available from the following companies:

Allergy Research Group
PRODUCT NAME: ThioDox™
CONTAINS: Lipoic Acid, NAC, and Glutathione, in tablet form

Source Naturals®
PRODUCT NAME: CHEM DEFENSE
Orange or peppermint in sublingual tablet form.

Carlson®
PRODUCT NAME: Glutathione Booster™
Available in capsule form

Prevail
PRODUCT NAME: GSH Cell Support
CONTAINS: Reduced L-Gluthathione and Anthocyanidins
Available in capsules

Grape Seed

Available from the following company:

Carlson®
PRODUCT NAME: Grape Seed extract: 130 MG
Available in softgel form

Herbs

Available from the following company:

Gaia Herbs, Inc.
PRODUCT NAME: Liquid Phyto-Caps™
A unique combination of superior bioavailability of a liquid extract with the convenience of a capsule.
For more information call 1-800-831-7780

Hawthorn

Available from the following company:

Prevail
PRODUCT NAME: Cardio Enzyme Formula
CONTAINS: Hawthorn Berry, Dan Shen Root, Arjun Bark, Passion Flower, Ginkgo
Available in capsules

Ipriflavone

Available from the following company:

Source Naturals®
PRODUCT NAME: ULTRA BONE BALANCE
CONTAINS: 600 mg of Ipriflavone, 1,200 mg Calcium, 600 mg Magnesium, as well as bone specific vitamins and minerals.

PRODUCT NAME: OSTIVONE
CONTAINS: Ipriflavone in tablet form.

Kava kava

Available from the following company:

Source Naturals®
PRODUCT NAME: KAVA PURE™ NUTRASPRAY

L-Carnitine

Available from the following company:

PRODUCT NAME: L-Carnitine 500
Sodium Free, available in 500mg capsules

Lutein

Available from the following company:

Solgar
PRODUCT NAME: Lutein Carotenoid Complex
Available in 15mg Vegicaps®

Lycopene

Available from the following companies:

Carlson®
PRODUCT NAME: Lycopene
Available in 5mg softgels

Source Naturals®
PRODUCT NAME: Lycopene
Antioxidant Carotenoid
Available in 5mg softgels

Magnesium

Available from the following companies:

Jarrow Formulas®
PRODUCT NAME: Magnesium Optimizer
CONTAINS: Magnesium Citrate, Potassium Chloride, and Taurine.
Available in Quik-Solv™ tablets

Source Naturals®
PRODUCT NAME: Magnesium Malate
Available in 1,000 mg tablet form.

MGN

Available from the following company:

Lane Labs
PRODUCT NAME: MGN 3 Ultra Immune Complex
CONTAINS: 250 mg of MGN-3 (rice bran enzymatically treated with shiitake mushroom extract), root fiber, calcium phosphate, silica, magnesium, serate, gelatin, water, glycerin.
Available in capsule form.

MSM

Available from the following companies:

Carlson®
PRODUCT NAME: MSM Sulfur
Each 1000mg capsule provides 334mg of organic sulfur

Jarrow Formulas™
PRODUCT NAME: MSM Sulfur™
Source of organic sulfur, available in 750mg capsules

Source Naturals®
PRODUCT NAME: MSM
CONTAINS: 1,500 mg MSM and 250 mg Vitamin C

Melatonin

Available from the following company:

Source Naturals®
PRODUCT NAME: Melatonin
Available in either 2.5 or 5mg sublingual tablet form in peppermint or orange flavor.

Multivitamin and Mineral Formulas—for Adults

Available from the following companies:

Carlson®
PRODUCT NAME: Super-1-Daily
In tablet form
Nutrients and excipients derived from sources other than animal, fish or fowl.
   Formulated to contain extra Vitamin B-12.

Prevail
PRODUCT NAME: Advance Multi-Vitamin and Minerals
Complete multi-vitamin with pure plant enzymes to enhance delivery and assimilation of
   nutrients
Available in capsules

Solgar
PRODUCT NAME: Omnium Multiple
A complete multiple including Alpha Lipoc Acid and Co-Q10.
Available in tablet form. Also available in iron and iodine free tablets

Source Naturals®
PRODUCT NAME: Life Force™ Multiple
Metabolic Activator, iron-free, in tablet form

Multivitamin and Mineral Formulas—for Children

Available from the following companies:

Prevail
PRODUCT: Children's Multi-Vitamin and Minerals
Complete multi-vitamin with pure plant enzymes to enhance deliery and assimilation of
   nutrients
Available in capsules

Carlson®
PRODUCT NAME: Scooter Rabbit
Chewable and tasty tablets containing 13 natural vitamins and 12 organic minerals.
   Sucrose-free.

Natrol®
PRODUCT NAME: My Favorite Multiple®
Available in capsules and tablets, also iron-free

Source Naturals®
PRODUCT NAME: Mega-Kid™
A delicious chewable multivitamin for children ages 1-10. Contains a full complement of vitamins and minerals, and also includes Bioflavanoids, Bee Pollen, Papaya and Rutin. See bottle for correct dosage according to age.

Mushrooms

Available from the following company:

Source Naturals®
PRODUCT NAME: Reishi Mushroom Supreme
Available in tablet form; 650mg.

PRODUCT NAME: Shitake Mushroom Supreme
Available in tablet form; 650mg.

N-Acetyl Cysteine

Available from the following companies:

Carlson®
PRODUCT NAME: N•A•C
Available in 500mg capsules

Solgar
PRODUCT NAME: NAC
Available in 600mg Vegicaps®

Olive Leaf Extract

Available from the following companies:

Natrol®
PRODUCT NAME: Olive Leaf Extract
Available in 610mg capsules

Nature's Plus
PRODUCT NAME: Herbal Actives
Standardized Olive Leaf Extract with 6% Oleuropein
Available in 250mg capsules

Source Naturals®
PRODUCT NAME: WELLNESS OLIVE LEAF
CONTAINS: Standarized extract yielding 75 mg of oleuropein in tablet form.

Poultry

Available from the following company:

Shelton's
Shelton's grows, processes and distributes free-range and antibiotic-free chickens and turkeys. For further information, call 1-800-541-1844

Probiotics (including Acidophilus)

Available from the following companies:

Allergy Research Group
PRODUCT NAME: ProGreens with Advanced Probiotic Formula
CONTAINS: organic gluten-free barley, wheat, alfalfa grasses, Spirulina, Chlorella
Dairy-free probiotic cultures
RECOMMENDED: 1 capsule per day

Jarrow Formulas™
PRODUCT NAME: Jarro-Dophilus™ + FOS
CONTAINS: 7 species, high potency, non-dairy probiotics. Hypoallergenic.
Available in capsule or powder form

Wakunaga
PRODUCT NAME: Kyo-Dophilus®
CONTAINS: L. acidophilus, B. bifidum, and B. longum, 1.5 billion live cells per capsule
RECOMMENDED: 1 capsule twice daily with meals

Pyconogenol™

Available from the following companies:

Henkel
Pycogenol® a pine bark extract supplying ingredients known as OPC's. Contains a complex of flavonoids and organic acids. Contact Henkel at 1-800-637-3702 for further information about this product and where it can be obtained.

Solgar Products
PRODUCT NAME: Pycnogenol® Capsules 30 mg
PRODUCT NAME: Pycnogenol® Vegicaps® 100 mg

Source Naturals
PRODUCT NAME: Pycnogenol®
Proanthocyanidin Complex
Available in 75 mg tablets

Quercetin

Available from the following companies:

Jarrow Formulas™
PRODUCT NAME: Quercetin 500™
Available in 500mg capsules

Source Naturals
PRODUCT NAME: Activated Quercetin
Non-allergenic Bioflavonoid Complex with Bromelain
Available in 1000mg tablets

PRODUCT NAME: Nutra Spray™ Quercetin
CONTAINS: Kava Root Extract 60 mg spray

Resveratrol

Available from the following companies:

Natrol®
PRODUCT NAME: Protykin™/Reservatrol
Available in capsules

Source Naturals®
PRODUCT NAME: Reservatrol
Available in 10mg tablets

Selenium

Available from the following companies:

Carlson®
PRODUCT NAME: Selenium
Available in 200mcg tablets

Natrol®
PRODUCT NAME: Selenium 200 Mcg
Available in 200mcg tablets

Source Naturals®
PRODUCT NAME: Selenomax®
High Selenium Yeast
Available in 200mcg tablets

Shark Cartilage

Available from the following company:

Lane Labs
PRODUCT NAME: Benefin® Shark Cartilage
CONTAINS: 750 mg of Benefin organically processed Shark Cartilage, carnauba wax, hypromellose, magnesium sterate, microcrystalline cellulose, tragacanth gum

Silymarin

Available from the following companies:

Jarrow Formulas™
PRODUCT NAME: Silymarin 80%
Standarized Milk Thistle 30:1 Concentrate, available in 150mg capsules

Source Naturals
PRODUCT NAME: Liver Guard
CONTAINS: CoQ10/N–Acetyl Cysteine Complex

St. John's Wort

Available through the following company:

Prevail
PRODUCT NAME: Hyperi-Max™
CONTAINS: St. John's Wort (0.3%), 5'HTP, Naicin, Siberian Ginseng
Available in capsules

Turmeric

Available from the following company:

Solgar
PRODUCT NAME: Turmeric Root Extract
CONTAINS: turmeric extract and raw turmeric powder
Available in 450mg Vegicaps®

Zinc

Available from the following companies:

Allergy Research Group
PRODUCT NAME: Zinc Citrate
Available in 25mg and 50mg capsules

PRODUCT NAME: Zinc Picolinate
Available in 25mg capsules

Jarrow Formulas™
PRODUCT NAME: Zinc Balance 15™
Zinc Monomethionate 15mg, Copper Gluconate 1mg, available in capsule form

Source Naturals®
PRODUCT NAME: Zinc
Amino Acid Chelate, 50mg

Special Resource Section

Bottled Spring Water

THE NEW SCIENCE OF WATER
Merlin: Merlin Water is twice purified to create a super pure water base. The source water is first purified through Reverse Osmosis and secondly purified with a proprietary process that further cleans the water removing heavy chemicals and dissolved contaminants. From this SuperPure water base, a special formulation of minerals and electrolytes are added back and electrochemically enhanced to create a mild alkalinity with antioxidant properties.

Merlin Water is available in glass and plastic packaging of 20 oz., 1.0 liter and bulk packaging of 4.0 liter and 18.0 liter in health food stores or by direct delivery. Call 1-800-982-2890 for further information or log onto *www.MERLINWATER.COM*.

Powdered Green Drinks

Available from the following companies:

Wakunaga of America Co., Ltd.
Kyo-Green® Powdered Drink Mix: A natural combination of young Barley and Wheat grasses blended with fine chlorella, brown rice and fine kelp. Available in health food stores. For more information, call 1-800-421-2998

Oncologics, Inc. (800-724-5566): Thera-Greens IPP contains over 50 ingredients, including antioxidants, phytonutricuts, and nutritional food extracts. Available in jars and capsules. Recommended: 2 scoops daily.

The Synergy Company™
Pure Synergy™, a certified organic superfood formula that is a blend of more than sixty of nature's finest and most potent superfoods-including 11 ocean and fresh water algae, 7 grass juices, 17 Chinese and 10 Western herbs, 5 immune supporting Asian mushrooms, plant enzymes, natural lecithin, royal jelly and natural anti-oxidants. Call 1-800-723-0277 for more information.

Fish

Crown Prince, Inc.: 800-255-5063 (all canned fish):
Brisling Sardines in Pure Olive Oil
Brisling Sardines in Water
Skinless & Boneless Sardines in Pure Olive Oil
Skinless & Boneless Sardines in Water
Pink Salmon
Albacore Tuna in Spring Water
Albacore Tuna in Spring Water—Low Sodium

Environmental Cleaning Products

Available from the following company:

Mountain Green™: Manutacturers of environmentally responsible household cleaning products without the use of harsh chemicals that harm the environment. Mountain Green is cruelty free and hypoallergenic.
Available products:

Ultra Liquid Laundry Detergent	32, 50 and 100 oz. bottles
Ultra Powdered Laundry Detergent	5.25 lb. box
Fabric Softener	32 oz. bottle
Non-cholorine bleach	32 oz. bottle
Natural Orange Dishwashing Liquid	22 oz. bottle
Natural Apple Dishwashing Liquid	22 oz. bottle
Automatic Diswasher Powder	4 lb. box
Glass Cleaner Spray	20 oz. bottle
All Purpose Cleaner Spray	20 oz. bottle
Multi-Purpose Degreaser Spray	20 oz. bottle

For further information regarding product availabliity, call 1-888-878-5781

Herbs

Chrysalis Natural Medicine Clinic & Herbal Pharmacy: Over 1,000 herbal medicines and nutrients from around the world, including hard-to-find Ayurvedic and Chinese herbs. (302-994-0565)

Gaia Herbs, Inc.: Producers of high quality liquid herbal extracts for over 12 years. Their recent development of liquid Phyto-Caps™ combines the superior bioavailability of a liquid extract with the convenience of a capsule. For the location of the nearest retail outlet or further information, call 1-800-831-7780.

Juicing Machine

Omega Products, Inc.: Omega's "New" Model 8000 Juicer with Twin Gears is designed to efficiently juice wheatgrass, carrots and most other fruits and vegetables. Runs at a low 90 rpms to retain the healthful enzymes needed for a healthy diet. Comes with a 5-year warranty.
(1-800-633-3401/717-561-1105)

Natural Cosmetics

Desert Essence: Vitamin E Therapy and other skin care products with Eco-Harvest Tea Tree Oil (888-476-8647)

Carlson® (800-323-4141)
E Gem Shampoo with Natural Vitamin E
E Gem Glycerine Soap with Vitamins E and A and no animal ingredients
ADE® Intensive Moisturizing Cream with Natural Vitamin E
Key•E® Moisturizing Cream with Natural Vitamin E
Key•E® Soothing Ointment with Natural Vitamin E

Oils (flax, olive oil, etc.)

Flora: Carries full line of organic oils, bottled in opaque glass, complete with pressing date.
Also carries UDO's CHOICE® PERFECTED OIL BLEND, an excellent balanced formula of omega-3, omega-6 and omega-9 fatty acids.
In United States, call 1-800-498-3610
In Canada, call 1-604-436-6000

Organic Foods

Goldmine Natural Food Company: Wide selection of hard-to-find organic grains, beans, and seeds; wheat-free pastas, soy products, sea products, sea vegetables, and Japanese green teas.
(1-800-475-3663/1-800-863-2347) *hhtp://www.goldminenaturalfood.com*

Tea Products

Guayaki Sustainable Rainforest Products, LLC: Producers of Organic, Shade-grown Yerba Mate, an energizing tea that is grown sustainably in the Paraguayan Rainforest. Available in tea bags and as a loose tea. Also available is a full line of alcohol-free whole plant liquid extracts (Peppermint, Lemongrass, Ginger, Cinnamon, Chai, Chamomile and Green Tea). For more information, call 1-888-GUAYAKI.

Wine

Frey Vineyards: Organic wines with no sulfites added. (1-800-760-3739)
Organic Wineworks: Producers of 100% organic wines. (1-800-699-9463) *http://www.organic.com*

There are also many high-quality, highly effective products that are marketed and sold only to health-care practitioners. These may not be available through your health-food store or mail-order suppliers. You can usually obtain these directly through your physician or health care practitioner.

Dr. Magaziner's Top Professional Line Nutritional Supplement Companies

ALLERGY RESEARCH GROUP
30806 Santana Street
Hayward, CA 94544
(510) 487-8526
(800) 545-9960
Fax (510) 487-8682
E-mail: *info@nutricology.com*
www.nutricology.com

DAVINCI LABORATORIES
20 New England Drive, C-1504
Essex Junction, VT 05453-1504
(800) 325-1776
(800) 878-5508
Fax (802) 878-0549
E-mail: *order@davincilabs.com*
www.davincilabs.com

DOUGLAS LABORATORIES®
600 Boyce Road
Pittsburg, PA 15205
(412) 494-0122
USA & Canada (800) 245-4440
or (888) DOUGLAB
Fax (412) 494-0155
Europe (31) (0) 455 444-7777
Fax Europe (31) (0) 455 44-55-33
E-mail: *nutrition@douglaslabs.com*
www.douglaslabs.com

ECOLOGICAL FORMULAS, INC.
CARDIOVASCULAR RESEARCH
1060 B Shary Circle
Concord, CA 94518
(800) 888-4585
(925) 827-2636
Fax (925) 676-9231
E-mail: *ecologicalformulas.com*

KLAIR LABORATORIES, INC.
140 Marine View Drive, Suite 110
Solana Beach, CA 92075
(760) 744-9680
(800) 533-7255
Fax (208) 665-2081
E-mail: *mail@aspenbenefits.com*
www.jymis.com\~david\development

LANE LABS
110 Commerce Drive
Allendale, NJ 07401
(800) 526-3005
(201) 236-9090 (Int'l)

METAGENICS
971 Calle Negocio
San Clemente, CA 92673
(949) 366-0818
(800) 692-9400
Fax (949) 366-2859
www.metagenics.net

PURE ENCAPSULATIONS®
490 Boston Post Road
Sudbury, MA 01776
(800) 753-CAPS
(978) 443-1999
Fax (888) 783-CAPS
www.pureencapsulations.com

THORNE RESEARCH, INC.
P.O. Box 25
Dover, ID 83825
(800) 228-1966
(208) 263-1337
Fax (800) 747-1950
E-mail: *info@thorne.com*
www.thorne.com

TYLER ENCAPSULATIONS
2204-8 N.W. Birdsdale
Gresham, OR 97030
USA (800) 869-9705
(503) 661-5401
Fax (503) 666-4913
E-mail: *info@tyler-inc.com*
www.tyler-inc.com

VITALINE FORMULAS
385 Williamson Way
Ashland, OR 97520
(800) 648-4755
(541) 482-9231
Fax (541) 482-9112
E-mail: *info@vitaline.com*
www.vitaline.com

"Allergy-Free" Products

You can check your local health-food store in order to find some of the allergy-free products, environmentally friendly products, and some of the nutritional supplements that were discussed earlier in this book. If you are unable to locate them, the following list will provide you with several mail-order companies to suit your needs. You can call them and request a catalog.

Allergy Research Shop 617-522-2795
Allergy Store 800-824-7163
American Environmental Health Foundation (AEHF) 800-428-2343
Environmental Health Shopper 800-447-1100
Environmental Purification Systems 415-682-7231
The Living Source 817-776-4878
National Ecological and Environmental Delivery System (N.E.E.D.S.) 800-634-1380

APPENDIX II

Reference Laboratories

As the field of nutritional biochemistry continues to advance, assessing your individual biochemical needs is rapidly becoming more sophisticated. I am often asked which laboratories I use to best assess a patient's nutrient balance, such as the levels of antioxidants, vitamins, trace minerals, toxic metals, amino acids, organic acids, essential fatty acids, hormones, viral load, adrenal or digestive disfunction, liver detoxification abilities, and other complex biochemical pathways. The following laboratories listed are those which I have found reliable and valuable in best assessing a patient's nutritional and biochemical status:

Dr. Magaziner's Top 10 Commercial Reference Laboratories Specializing in Nutritional Biochemistry

AccuChem Laboratories
990 N. Bowser Road
Suite 880
Richardson, TX 75081
800-451-0116
FAX: 972-234-6095
www.accuchemlabs.com

AAL Reference Laboratories, Inc.
1715 E. Wilshire #715
Santa Ana, CA 92705
800-522-2611
FAX: 714-543-2034
www.antibodyassay.com

Diagnos-Techs, Inc.
6620 S. 192nd Place, Building J
Kent, WA 98032
800-878-3787
FAX: 425-251-0637

Doctors Data, Inc.
3755 Illinois Avenue
St. Charles, IL 60174
800-323-2784
FAX: 630-587-7860
www.doctorsdata.com

Great Smokies Diagnostic Laboratory
63 Zillicoa Street
Asheville, NC 28801-1074
800-522-4762
FAX: 828-252-9303
www.greatsmokies-lab.com

ImmunoLaboratories, Inc.
1620 W. Oakland Park Boulevard
Fort Lauderdale, FL 33311
800-231-9197
FAX: 305-739-6563
www.immunolabs.com

Immunosciences Lab, Inc.
8730 Wilshire Boulevard, Suite 305
Beverly Hills, CA 90211
800-950-4686
FAX: 310-657-1053
E-mail: *immunsci@ix.netcom.com*
www.immuno-sci-lab.com

Spectracell Laboratories, Inc.
515 Post Oak Boulevard, Suite 830
Houston, TX 77027-9409
800-227-5227
FAX: 713-621-3234
E-mail: *spec1@spectracell.com*
www.spectracell.com

MetaMetrix Clinical Laboratory
5000 Peachtree Ind. Boulevard
Norcross, GA 30071
800-221-4640
FAX: 770-441-2237
www.metametrix.com

The Great Plains Laboratory
9335 W. 75th Street
Overland Park, KS 66204
913-341-8949
FAX: 913-341-6207
www.greatplainslaboratory.com

Compounding Pharmacies

Compounding pharmacies have been an invaluable asset to physicians specializing in alternative and complimentary medicine. With a physician's prescription, these pharmacies can prepare specialized formulations such as customized medications or nutritional supplements that are hypoallergenic, free of food colorings, dye, or sugar, or produce products with unique delivery system and dosages. The following is a list of compounding pharmacies who are likely to meet your needs.

Dr. Magaziner's Top 10 Compounding Pharmacies

ApotheCure
13720 Midway Road
Suite 109
Dallas, TX 75244
800-969-6601
FAX: 800-687-5252

Hazel Drugs Apothecary
Compounding Pharmacy
20 N. Laurel Street
Hazelton, PA 18201
800-439-2026
FAX: 800-400-8764
www.hazeldrugs.com

College Pharmacy
3505 Austin Bluffs Parkway
Suite 101
Colorado Springs, CO 80918
800-888-9358
FAX: 800-556-5893
www.collegepharmacy.com

Hopewell Pharmacy and Compounding Center
1 W. Broad Street
Hopewell, NJ 08534
800-792-6670
FAX: 609-466-8222
www.hopewellrx.com

Key Pharmacy
23422 Pacific Highway South
Kent, WA 98032
800-878-1322
FAX: 206-878-1114

Lakeside Pharmacy
4632 Highway 58
Chattanooga, TN 37416
800-523-1486
FAX: 877-890-8435
www.lakesidepharmacy.com

Medical Center Compounding Pharmacy
3675 S. Rainbow Boulevard, #103
Las Vegas, NV 89103
800-723-7455
FAX: 800-238-8239
www.mccpharmacy.com

Professional Arts Pharmacy
1101 N. Rolling Road
Baltimore, MD 21228
800-832-9285
FAX: 888-663-5686
E-mail: *mortlpestl@aol.com*

Wellness Health & Pharmaceuticals
2800 S. 18th Street
Birmingham, AL 35209
800-227-2627
FAX: 800-369-0302
E-mail: *wellness@e-pages.com*
www.wellnesshealth.com

Women's International Pharmacy
5708 Monona Drive
Madison, WI 53716-3152
800-279-5708
FAX: 800-279-8011

APPENDIX III

Professional Organizations

In order to find more information on any of the topics discussed in this book or to find a qualified health-care practitioner who emphasizes wellness and natural healing techniques, you may contact any of the following professional organizations:

American Academy of Environmental
   Medicine (AAEM)
American Financial Center
7701 East Kellogg, Suite 625
Wichita, KS 67207-1705
Phone: 316-684-5500
Fax: 316-684-5709

American Association of Naturopathic
   Physicians (AANP)
601 Valley Street, Suite 105
Seattle, WA 98109
Phone: 206-298-0215
Fax: 206-298-0129
E-mail: *webmaster@naturopathic.org*

American Association of Oriental Medicine
   (AAOM)
433 Front Street
Catasauqua, PA 18032
Phone: 610-266-1433
Fax: 610-264-2768
E-mail: *aaom1@aol.com*

American Botanical Counsel (ABC)
PO Box 201660
Austin, TX 78720
Phone: 800-373-7105
Fax: 512-331-1924

American Chiropractic Association
1701 Clarendon Boulevard
Arlington, VA 22209
Phone: 800-986-INFO
Fax: 703-243-2593
E-mail: *info@amerchiro.org*

American College for Advancement in
   Medicine (ACAM)
23121 Verdugo Drive, Suite 204
Laguna Hills, CA 92653
Phone: 800-532-3688
Fax: 949-455-9679
E-mail: *acam@acam.org*

American Holistic Medical Association
   (AHMA)
6728 Old McLean Village Drive
McLean, VA 22101-3906
Phone: 703-556-9728
Fax: 703-566-8729
E-mail: *HolistMed@aol.com*

American Massage Therapy Association
   (AMTA)
820 David Street, Suite 100
Evanston, IL 60201-4444
Phone: 847-864-0123
Fax: 847-864-1178
E-mail: *info@inet.amtamassage.org*

American Preventive Medical Association
(APMA)
PO Box 458
Great Falls, VA 22066
Phone: 800-230-APMA
Fax: 703-759-6711
E-mail: *apma@healthy.net*

American Society for Clinical Hypnosis
(ASCH)
2200 East Devon Avenue, Suite 291
Des Plaines, IL 60018
Phone: 847-297-3317
Fax: 847-297-7309
E-mail: *70632.1663@compuserve.com*

American Yoga Association
PO Box 19986
Sarasota, FL 34276
Phone: 941-953-5859
Fax: 941-364-9153

Biofeedback Certification Institute of
America (BCIA)
10200 W. 44th Avenue, Suite 304
Wheat Ridge, CO 80033-2840
Phone: 303-420-2902
Fax: 303-422-3394

Foundation for the Advancement of
Innovative Medicine (FAIM)
485 Kinderkamack Road, 2nd Floor
Oradell, NJ 07649
Phone: 877-634-3246
Fax: 201-634-1871
E-mail: *faim@fcc.net*
www.faim.org

Herb Research Foundation
1007 Pearl Street, Suite 200
Boulder, CO 80302
Phone: 303-449-2265
Fax: 303-449-7849

Homeopathic Educational Services
2124 Kittredge Street
Berkeley, CA 94704
Phone: 510-649-0294
Fax: 510-649-1955
E-mail: *mail@homeopathic.com*

International Foundation for Homeopathy
2366 Eastlake Avenue East, Suite 325
Seattle, WA 98102
Phone: 425-776-4147
Fax: 425-776-1499

National Acupuncture and Oriental
Medicine Alliance
14637 Starr Road, SE
Olalla, WA 98359
Phone: 253-851-6896
Fax: 253-851-6883

National Center for Homeopathy
801 North Fairfax Street, Suite 306
Alexandria, VA 22314
Phone: 703-548-7790
Fax: 703-548-7792
E-mail: *nchinfo@igc.apc.org*

National Certification Commission for
  Acupuncture and Oriental Medicine
  (NCCAOM)
11 Canal Center Plaza
Suite 300
Alexandria, VA 22314
Phone: 703-548-9004
Fax: 703-548-9079
E-mail: *info@nccaom.org*

Price-Pottenger Nutrition Foundation
PO Box 2614
La Mesa, CA 90943
Phone: 800-FOODS 4 YOU
Fax: 619-574-1314
E-mail: *info@price-pottenger.org*

Magaziner Center for Wellness and Anti-Aging Medicine

General Philosophy

The philosophy of the Magaziner Center for Wellness and Anti-Aging Medicine is to prevent disease and to promote optimum health. We strive to achieve this through integrating modern medical care with the latest advances in nutrition and preventive medicine.

The most recent medical evidence supports our clinical approach—stressing the vital role of proper nutrition in maintaining good health and preventing disease. Our approach focuses on natural, nontoxic means of treatment. Although medications are prescribed when necessary, our treatment emphasizes natural therapies utilizing vitamins, minerals, enzymes, amino acids, herbs, botanicals, and homeopathics.

We use the latest state-of-the-art technology and laboratory testing to best access your body's biochemistry. Through comprehensive biochemical analysis of blood, saliva, urine, and stool, we can identify allergies and nutritional health problems. We are then able to design a comprehensive individualized program for your personal needs.

All health conditions benefit from treatment at the Magaziner Center in Cherry Hill, New Jersey. The integration of our unique, comprehensive, and individualized approach has had remarkable results. For more than a decade, our programs have helped thousands of people with a variety of disorders.

Some of the Conditions Successfully Treated Include:

Adrenal dysfunction	Colitis and digestive disorders	Macular degeneration
Allergies		Menopausal symptoms
Arthritis	Coronary heart disease	Mental toxicity
Asthma	Depression and anxiety	Musculoskeletal problems
Autism	Diabetes	Obesity
Cancer	Fibromyalgia	Osteoporosis
Candida yeast syndrome	Hormone problems	Premenstrual syndrome
Cholesterol problems	Hypertension	Prostate disorders
Chronic fatigue	Hypoglycemia	Sinusitis
Chronic headaches	Immune dysfunction	Skin disorders
Chronic infections	Irritable bowel syndrome	Stroke
Chronic vaginitis	Learning disorders and ADD	

The Magaziner Center for Wellness and Anti-Aging Medicine provides comprehensive medical management for achieving optimum health.

Evaluations and Treatment Modalities Include:
Natural healing
Allergy treatment
Environmental medicine
Nutritional medicine
Preventive medicine
Chelation and Intravenous therapy
Cancer prevention/treatment
Prolotherapy
Homeopathy
Anti-Aging Medicine
Stress Reduction

Magaziner Center for Wellness and Anti-Aging Medicine
1907 Greentree Road
Cherry Hill, NJ 80003-1112
Tel: 856-424-8222
Fax: 856-424-2599
E-mail: *info@drmagaziner.com*
www.drmagaziner.com

At the Magaziner Center, we offer a free telephone health hotline where a member of the staff is always available to answer your health questions. Call any Tuesday or Wednesday between 5 and 6 P.M. to speak to one of our physicians.

Hotline (Free information): 856-424-0707

INDEX

minerals, 8–11
 important minerals, their functions,
  sources, and effects of deficiency,
  9–11
 losses in flour refining, 83
 mineral deficiencies, 172
modifying diet and lifestyle, 3
mold, 154, 157–58
monounsaturated fats, 46, 53
morning sickness, 266
multiple chemical sensitivity (MCS),
 162
multiple sclerosis (MS), 266–67

National Academy of Sciences, 162
National Aeronautics & Space
 Administration (NASA), 169
natural therapies, treating common illnesses naturally, 219–78
neurotransmitters, 191
nicotinamide adenine dinucleotide
 (NADH), 209
nondairy foods, 25
nori, 77, 78
NutriSweet®, 44
nutrition labels. *See* food labels

obesity, 267–68
 glycemic index and, 119
octacosanol, 209
olive leaf extract, 209–10
 omega-3 fatty acids
 cod liver oil, 205
 DHA, 205
 fish oils, 206
 flaxseed oil, 206
 omega-3 oils (alpha-linolenic acid),
  55
omega-6 oils (linoleic acid), 55
osteoarthritis, 226–27
osteoporosis, 264, 268–70
oxalate, 117
oxalic acid, 117

pangamic acid, 205
Paracelsus, 57
partially hydrogenated fats, 46, 50
personal products, 173–74
pesticides, 161
petrochemicals, 167
pharmacies, compounding, 311–12
phenol, 167
phenylalanine, 44
phosphatidylserine (PS), 210
phytochemicals, 17
plants
 plant-based foods, 27, 28
 and their protection against pollution, 169
pollens, 153, 154, 155–56
polyphenols, 207

polyunsaturated fats, 46, 50, 53
potassium, 11
 diuretics and depletion of, 19
premenstrual syndrome (PMS), 270
proanthocyanidins (PCOs), 207, 210
professional organizations, 314–316
propionibacterium acnes, 220
propolis, bee pollen and, 204
prostaglandins, 55
prostate enlargement, 271–72
protease, 32
proteins, amino acids, and enzymes,
 27
 amino acids, 30–31
 combinations for forming complete
  proteins, 29
 enzymes, 32
 getting protein without eating meat,
  29
 glutathione, 33
 proteins, 27–28
psoriasis, 272–73
purines, 118
Pycnogenol®, 210

Qi, 193–94
quercetin, 210

reactive hypoglycemia, 108
red yeast rice, 210–11
Reishi mushrooms, 212
relaxation therapies, 192–93
resveratrol, 211
rheumatoid arthritis, 226–28
rolfing, 194
rosacea, 273–74
rotation diet, 97–100
Russell, Bertrand, 191

S-adenosyl-methionin (SAMe), 211
saccharin, 44
safer alternatives, 173
 cleaning agents, 175–76
 insecticides, 178–79
 personal products, 173–74
salicylates, 114–16
SAMe, 211
saturated fats, 46, 53
sea vegetables, 75–78
seaweed, 75
shark cartilage, 211
shiatzu, 193–94
Shiitake mushrooms, 212
sick-building syndrome, 163
simple sugars, 35
sinus infections, 274–75
skin disorders
 eczema, 248–49
 psoriasis, 272–73
 rosacea, 273–74
smoking, 90

sodium bisulfite, 87
soluble fiber, 68
sore throat, 275
soy products, 27–28
Staphylococcus aureus, 230
Stevia, 43
sucralose, 43
sugar. *See* carbohydrates and sugars
sulfites, 87
sulfur dioxide, 87
super nutrients, 203–12
superoxide dismutase (SOD), 32
supplements. *See* vitamins

T-helper cells, 209
tocotrienols, 212
trans-fatty acids, 50

ulcers, 276

varicose veins, 277
vegetarian diet
 lower cholesterol levels, 63
 protein needs and vegetarian foods,
  29
 soy products and vegetarian cooking, 28
vision problems
 catatacts, 236–37
 glaucoma, 255
 macular degeneration, 263
vital nutrients, 3
 anticancer produce, 16
 antioxidants, 13–15
 calcium, 25–26
 medications and depletion of nutrients, 19–24
 minerals, 8–11
 phytochemicals, 17
 vegetables, 18–19
 vitamins, 5–8
 what's wrong with the American
  diet?, 4
vitamins, 5
 factors that make taking nutritional
  supplements necessary, 12
 losses in flour refining, 83
 major vitamins, their functions,
  sources, and effects of deficiency, 6–8
 natural vs. synthetic, 12–13
 supplement companies, 285–308
 vitamin deficiencies, 172
 who needs supplements?, 12

wakame, 77, 78
water, 176
 water filters, 176
 water purification systems, 176–77
water-soluble vitamins, 5
weight-loss diet, 112

ABOUT THE AUTHOR

Dr. Allan Magaziner is a nationally acclaimed medical expert on health and nutrition related topics and the therapeutic effects of nutritional supplements. He has been on numerous television programs, cited by prestigious magazines, and has been a quoted authority for books and newspaper articles throughout the United States. He has been a popular and much sought-after presenter for numerous medical organizations, hospitals, medical schools, colleges, universities, and lay public groups, educating them on the practical applications and rationale for therapeutic nutrition.

Dr. Magaziner is also the author of the best seller *The Complete Idiot's Guide to Living Longer and Healthier*. Dr. Magaziner's easy-to-read books provide comprehensive and practical modalities for improving your health. His books blend the accumulation of nearly twenty years of clinical experience in successfully treating thousands of patients, along with the latest research supporting advances in alternative and complementary medicine.

Dr. Magaziner has completed a fellowship in allergy and environmental medicine as well as postgraduate training in clinical nutrition and preventive medicine. He is a distinguished member of the Board of Directors and Fellow of the American College for Advancement in Medicine. He is also their Vice President and National Program Chairman. Dr. Magaziner holds Board Certifications in Family Practice, Environmental Medicine and Chelation Therapy. He is the founder and medical director of the prestigious Magaziner Center for Wellness and Anti-Aging Medicine in Cherry Hill, New Jersey.